Mental Health Medications for Children

The Guilford Practical Intervention in the Schools Series

Kenneth W. Merrell, Series Editor

Books in this series address the complex academic, behavioral, and social–emotional needs of children and youth at risk. School-based practitioners are provided with practical, research-based, and readily applicable tools to support students and team successfully with teachers, families, and administrators. Each volume is designed to be used directly and frequently in planning and delivering clinical services. Features include a convenient format to facilitate photocopying, step-by-step instructions for assessment and intervention, and helpful, timesaving reproducibles.

Mental Health Medications for Children

A Primer

RONALD T. BROWN
LAURA ARNSTEIN CARPENTER
EMILY SIMERLY

Foreword by Martin T. Stein, MD

THE GUILFORD PRESS
New York   London

To those who have taught me and mentored me along the way, and to Marti Hagan, whose support and efforts have made it possible to get there.
—R. T. B.

To Donna and Walter Arnstein, for their love and support.
—L. A. C.

To my brother, Dr. Terry Simerly, who has always led the way, and to Marti Hagan, who got me into all this to start with.
—E. S.

© 2005 The Guilford Press
A Division of Guilford Publications, Inc.
72 Spring Street, New York, NY 10012
www.guilford.com

Printed in Canada

This book is printed on acid-free paper.

Last digit is print number: 9 8 7 6 5 4 3 2 1

Library of Congress Cataloging-in-Publication Data
Brown, Ronald T.
    Mental health medications for children: a primer / Ronald T. Brown, Laura Arnstein Carpenter, and Emily Simerly.
        p. cm.—(The Guilford practical intervention in the schools series)
    Includes bibliographical references and index.
    ISBN 1-59385-202-9
    1. Pediatric psychopharmacology. I. Carpenter, Laura Arnstein. II. Simerly, Emily. III. Title. IV. Series.
    RJ504.7.B766 2005
    615.′78′083—dc22
                                                                    2005001601

About the Authors

Ronald T. Brown, PhD, ABPP, is Professor of Public Health, Pediatrics, and Psychology, and Dean of the College of Health Professions at Temple University. Currently editor of the *Journal of Pediatric Psychology*, he has published several books and over 200 articles and chapters in the areas of pediatric psychology and pediatric psychopharmacology. Dr. Brown was formerly President of the Society for Pediatric Psychology and currently serves the National Institutes of Health, Center for Scientific Review, study section on behavioral medicine interventions and outcomes. He is a diplomate in Clinical Health Psychology of the American Board of Professional Psychology and a fellow in the American Psychological Association, the American Psychological Society, and the National Academy of Neuropsychology.

Laura Arnstein Carpenter, PhD, is Assistant Professor of Pediatrics at the Medical University of South Carolina. Dr. Carpenter is a licensed clinical psychologist specializing in the assessment and treatment of autism spectrum disorders, and has extensive training and clinical experience in pediatric neuropsychology. She has cowritten nine articles and chapters, and has made more than 30 presentations at regional and national scientific conferences.

Emily Simerly, PhD, is Clinical Director of the Mental Health Unit at the Georgia Diagnostic and Classification Prison in Jackson, Georgia, a maximum security men's intake prison that also houses Death Row. She is also Regional Clinical Director of mental health units at a number of prisons in northern Georgia. Dr. Simerly has published articles in *Voices* and has written a chapter in *Psychotherapy and the Poverty Patient*. As a clinician, she uses a humanistic–existential foundation to practice in-depth psychotherapy, using many cognitive behavioral techniques.

Foreword

As a pediatrician, I am in the forefront of the evaluation and treatment of children and adolescents with a variety of conditions that affect learning, emotional development, and social interactions. When we pediatricians consider common conditions such as attention-deficit/hyperactivity disorder and depression or less common conditions such as autism and psychosis, we are aware that we cannot work alone. Other professionals are critical to the development of the correct diagnosis and to monitoring treatment, and often provide behavioral management, classroom accommodations, and other forms of therapy. Parents (and other caretakers) and school professionals are our most important allies in helping children with all behavioral conditions.

Ronald T. Brown and his colleagues have written a comprehensive and practical guide to helping nonphysicians understand medications—how they work, when they are prescribed, how to consider risks versus benefits, and how to monitor the effects and side effects of medications. There are so many practical suggestions in each chapter that I found myself taking notes to share with my colleagues, students, and office staff.

The content of the book is directed at teachers, school administrators, school psychologists, nurses, parents, and grandparents. I would extend the list of those who might find useful information in this book to include others who work with children in a variety of activities, including youth group leaders, camp counselors, scout leaders, and those who teach outside the usual classroom (music teachers, dance instructors, sports coaches, and religious teachers). Considering the growing number of children and adolescents taking medications for psychological disorders today, everyone who interacts with these children will benefit from the knowledge in this book.

The chapters comprise a pharmacology text for those who have not studied medicine or psychiatry. Each section is written in clear language. When technical terms are used, the authors are careful to define the term and place it in the context of a particular condition. A glossary of medical and psychological terms is included, and there are numerous, easy-to-read tables of medications and mental health conditions in each chapter.

The reader is encouraged to use the material in the book as an introduction to medications, and the authors provide suggestions for ongoing learning through the available media. Chapter 1, "Overview and Pediatric Psychopharmacology Practices," is an excellent discussion of medicines that affect children's brains. The reader learns about the way these medicines affect neuroreceptors (i.e., which transfer information from one nerve to another in the brain), the cautious approval process by the U.S. Food and Drug Administration, the importance of monitoring drug effects and side effects, and the myth of addiction (for most prescribed medications). The educational and social benefits of medications for specific conditions are described. Teachers and other school personnel are provided with suggestions for improving adherence to medications.

Chapter 2 is entitled "The Importance of School Personnel on the Treatment Team." It took me many years to appreciate the significance of this statement. Teachers are a critical part of the diagnostic and treatment team. The authors have come up with a long list of creative strategies for communicating with parents (e.g., be specific when talking to parents about a child's behavior by describing the actual behavior rather than using general or technical terms) and with physicians (a letter from a teacher to a physician is provided in Appendix 3 as an example). They offer guidelines for talking to a parent who is resistant to using medications for his or her child (suggesting behavioral alternatives and information about medications) and for helping a child who is anxious or embarrassed to leave the classroom to take medication.

Knowledge about medications that improve behavior, learning, and social interactions does not have to be highly technical. The authors have demystified the field of "psychopharmacology" in Chapter 3. An up-to-date review of frequently prescribed and less frequently prescribed medications will give teachers and other readers a concise and comprehensive overview of these medications. Clear writing and the use of well-planned tables ease the learning process. Chapter 4 expands the medication information by linking specific drugs with psychiatric and learning-related disorders. The reader appreciates that there are often several types of medication available for each condition. Different benefits and different adverse side effects guide a physician to use one medication or another. School personnel will learn why a medication is prescribed, the target behaviors shown to be improved with a particular medication, and the alternatives available when the medication does not work effectively or produces intolerable side effects. Case examples are plentiful and are all real-world experiences that illustrate the monitoring process of children taking medications. These chapters will produce a better-informed teacher when communicating with parents and physicians as part of the treatment team. I suspect they will also have a positive effect on teaching these children and others in the classroom. In Chapter 5 there are numerous suggestions on useful ways to monitor treatment in the school. Behavior observation logs and a method of charting behaviors are provided with case examples. There is an excellent discussion of the placebo effect found in all medical therapies.

Mental Health Medications for Children: A Primer is an outstanding book written by knowledgeable professionals with practical experience in providing care and working with school personnel and parents of children with a variety of mental health conditions. This book should appeal to a wide audience, particularly to those educators who participate in the growth and development of children with challenging behavioral conditions. We needed this book a long time ago, but it's not too late!

Martin T. Stein, MD
Director of Developmental–Behavioral Pediatrics
University of California at San Diego
Children's Hospital San Diego

Preface

The model of care for children presented in this book is a treatment team model that involves all professionals and others who provide information that improves the care of a child. Researchers and clinicians have shown time and time again that the more information available for making treatment decisions, the better those decisions will be. In this book, we strive to find the best care for children through the inclusion of significant caregivers.

As teachers, school psychologists, nurses, school administrators, and others, you work for a school system with guidelines and standard operating procedures that usually address communication among teachers, parents, and other professionals involved in the care of schoolchildren. Please familiarize yourself with those guidelines so you can discern the appropriate course of action to relay your concern about children in your care.

In most states, physicians are the primary prescribers of medication. They regularly read journals and online publications with information on recent advances, innovative methods, and drugs available for the problems they are treating. The data provided by other members of the treatment team are invaluable in helping the physician or other primary provider arrive at the best choices for care.

Anyone who reads the news or watches television is aware of the rapidly changing data about medications and the science surrounding them. New findings can quickly make previously rock-solid information become obsolete. We encourage you to keep up with changes in medical practice. Newspapers in larger cities usually have articles about new findings. Many newspapers, including *The New York Times*, are available online for free. The Internet is a resource with limitless information. Consumer advocate groups like the National Alliance for the Mentally Ill maintain websites with a considerable amount of information and ideas. Another website is WebMD, which provides good basic information on many mental illnesses. These media will keep you up to date and better able to help your students.

Support groups are usually thought of as being for parents of children diagnosed with a disorder. However, as a school professional, you can learn much from these groups, which offer many ideas for treatment plans. You might start a support group among your peers and consider it a peer supervision group.

Remember, you are an integral person in the treatment of children with psychiatric disorders. We hope this book is helpful to you as you work to help your students and their families.

ACKNOWLEDGMENTS

We would like to express our appreciation to the staff of The Guilford Press for their guidance and patience. We would also like to acknowledge the able and steady editorial and other skills of Word Wizards in bringing this book to print. Finally, we thank Pat W. Wells, LaDonna Benedict, Kelly Stone, Franklin Abbot, Barbara Locascio, Jill Kneuppel, and Craig Storlie for comments on earlier versions of several of the chapters.

Contents

1

Overview and Pediatric Psychopharmacology Practices

WHY A BOOK ABOUT MEDICATIONS FOR SCHOOLCHILDREN?

Children, it is said, are our most precious resource. If this is true, then it is incumbent upon us to provide them the very best care possible. Our idea for writing this book stemmed from our belief that the knowledge and experience we can provide to you can help children receive the care that will create a better next generation. We wanted to help those who are on the frontlines every day—teachers, school administrators, school psychologists, nurses, parents, and grandparents—make the myriad daily decisions that go into forming a healthy child.

Raising children in the world today is a very complex task that gets more complex with each passing year. We created this book to serve as a reference guide for understanding and working with school-age children and adolescents. We are also aware that the book could be useful and of benefit to a larger circle of others who have crucial input into the welfare of children. Thus, we designed the book primarily for school personnel but invite others to use it as it is helpful.

Our book provides an overview of the use of medications for learning, mood, and behavior for school-age children. It should be useful for individuals working in special education and regular education settings. We have written this book for individuals who may have not been trained in psychopharmacology. Whenever possible, we will replace technical terms with more common ones, and we will explain the logic of medical jargon. For additional assistance and because many of the terms used in the book may be new to some readers, a glossary is provided at the end of the book.

Structure

The use of medications by children and adolescents in schools is reviewed in Chapter 1. A section is devoted to basic terminology associated with psychopharmacology. In Chapter 2 we discuss issues related to medication use in children, including the importance of adherence to treatment and legal and ethical concerns. We also present effective strategies for communicating with medical professionals. There are two ways to organize information about psychopharmacology, and these are described in Chapters 3 and 4. In Chapter 3, we discuss the major types (classes) of medications. We also describe the cognitive and behavioral effects associated with each medication. This chapter is a quick reference to information about specific medications.

Chapter 4 provides an overview of various psychiatric disorders in children and adolescents and describes the types of medications that are used to manage these disorders. In Chapter 5, we describe methods to monitor the effects of treatment, and we describe adverse side effects. The appendices contain helpful, reproducible tables and forms.

Objectives

We designed this book to help you:

- Navigate medication use.
- Recognize and understand basic terms and concepts in pharmacology.
- Understand how various medications affect the brain.
- Identify classifications of the major psychotropic agents used with children and adolescents.
- Be aware of the way medications affect how children think, feel, and behave.
- Learn common childhood psychiatric disorders and the medications that are most often used in their management.
- Communicate effectively with physicians and parents to offer important information and help guide treatment choices.
- Be familiar with ethical and legal issues surrounding the use of medications with school-age children.

Importance

The following case histories describe some of the challenges facing today's parents, teachers and teachers' aides, principals, school nurses, coaches, and school support staff.

Ramon is an 8-year-old boy with attention-deficit/hyperactivity disorder (ADHD). He takes his medication before he comes to school in the morning and usually is a very good student. Lately, his teacher has noticed that he has often been talking out of turn. He has missed recess 3 days in the last week due to problem behavior. His school performance has been slipping.

1. Should you ask Ramon if he has been taking his medication?
2. What is the best way to communicate your concerns with Ramon's parents and physician?
3. Could these behaviors be related to his medications?
4. What should you say if other children ask about Ramon's behavior?

Stephanie is an 11-year-old girl with a long history of epilepsy. She takes medication at home and at school to manage seizures. Lately, Stephanie has seemed very drowsy during class and has been having problems concentrating on her work.

1. What are some common side effects of the medication Stephanie is taking?
2. What else could be causing Stephanie to behave this way?
3. Could these behaviors be a sign of a very serious problem? Do you need to take immediate action or can the issue wait until the parent–teacher conference?
4. Must Stephanie take her medication at the same time every day? What should you do if she misses a dose?

Evan is a 5-year-old boy who is starting school for the first time. He has a hard time remembering to raise his hand before talking or standing up. He seems to be constantly on the go, and it seems impossible for him to stay in a chair during brief work sessions. He always seems to be in time-out.

1. How should you communicate your concerns to Evan's parents?
2. What kind of information can you provide to Evan's physician to help make the best decisions about his diagnosis and treatment?
3. If Evan is prescribed medication, what kind of feedback should teachers provide the physician and parents about his behavior?
4. If Evan is prescribed medication, how can you help him with difficult feelings when the other kids find out?

Malika is a 14-year-old girl with autism and mental retardation. Although she is making good progress at school, she bangs her head against her desk and other hard surfaces and screams loudly whenever her routine is disrupted. You know that she is taking medication to treat symptoms of hyperactivity, impulsivity, and inattention, and you know she occasionally refuses to take the medication. You wonder if a different or additional treatment approach might be helpful to the adolescent.

1. What is the best way for teachers to provide information about Malika's behavior to her parents and physician?
2. Is it appropriate for teachers to talk to Malika's parents and physicians about their concerns about her medication?
3. What side effects are associated with her current medication?
4. Is it dangerous for her to miss a dose of her current medication?

Ramon, Stephanie, Evan, and Malika are only a few examples of the reasons an increasing number of schoolchildren are taking psychotropic medications. Daily administration of psychotropic medication to children and adolescents creates numerous practical, ethical, and legal concerns for school professionals. What symptoms should the medications target? What side effects are associated with the medication? Which side effects are dangerous and warrant immediate attention? When should a teacher tell a parent that the child might need medication? How can school professionals help children who take medications to develop healthy attitudes about their treatments? How can they smooth the way for children to fit in with their peers? These questions are not casual or philosophical but relate to the daily experiences of those who provide care for children in school.

Professionals who have experience with school-age children probably have noticed that more children seem to be taking medication today than ever before. Unfortunately, no national database exists yet to provide comprehensive information on how many children receive specific psychotropic medications for specific problems. However, recent surveys indicate that these medications are now being prescribed more frequently to pediatric populations (Vitiello, 2001). According to one survey, about 6% of schoolchildren were receiving medication for management of symptoms of ADHD. Younger children were more likely to be taking medication than older children with this disorder. In this survey, third graders were the most likely to be receiving medication.

Boys are five times more likely to receive treatment for ADHD than girls (Safer & Krager, 1988). Although children are most likely to receive stimulant treatment (the treatment of choice for ADHD) during elementary school, it is becoming increasingly common for children to continue treatment for ADHD into high school and even adulthood.

Medications are also increasingly being prescribed for children with other disorders. About one-third of individuals with autism take some form of psychotropic medication, often a stimulant or an antipsychotic (Aman, Van Bourgondien, Wolford, & Sarphare, 1995). About 5% of schoolchildren and adolescents with mental retardation receive medication (Gadow, 1993). These percentages go much higher for children in residential facilities. Antidepressants are also being prescribed more frequently for children with a variety of disorders, not just depression (Emslie, Mays, & Hughes, 2000).

Some people have questioned whether medications are being overused for certain conditions. In particular, are children with ADHD being prescribed medication instead of receiving proper behavioral interventions that have less impact on their physical health? Are medications a short-term substitute for necessary school reform? Safer, Zito, and Fine (1996) found children from low socioeconomic backgrounds were, at best, receiving about the same prescriptions for stimulant medications as children from more affluent neighborhoods. Perl (1992) found that children from more affluent areas were more likely to have prescriptions for ADHD, which indicated that, at least in Perl's sample of children, affluent children were more likely to be medicated than poor children. Race as a factor has also been studied. Hispanic and African American children were prescribed stimulants less often than Caucasian children (Fox, Foster, & Zito, 2000). These findings seem to say that children with access to the best medical care and schools are the most likely to receive treatment. They also give some indication that minority and less affluent children do not seem to be overmedicated compared to affluent children and perhaps may be receiving less than optimal consideration for medication.

BENEFITS OF PSYCHOTROPIC MEDICATIONS FOR CHILDREN

An important question is whether medications can make meaningful changes in a child's life. There are numerous individual stories of how children have been helped by medications, and researchers who have studied large samples of children have also come to the same conclusion. Medications can have significant beneficial effects for children's learning, behavior, and quality of life. The area most researched has been treatment effects of stimulant medication for children with ADHD, although findings likely extend to children with a wide range of emotional, behavioral, and learning problems. It seems that stimulant medication can significantly reduce symptoms of hyperactivity and inattention in children with ADHD. Reductions of these problems can lead to educational benefits, including:

- Improved capacity to benefit from educational interventions.
- Better attention and concentration on tasks.
- More accurate performance on academic tasks.
- Faster performance on academic tasks.
- Less time spent on consequences for misbehavior (e.g., less time in time-out).

In addition to educational benefits, stimulant medication provides dramatic social benefits. The medicine, when prescribed and monitored properly, affects not only the way the child behaves but also the way the world behaves toward the child. When the child is treated differently and more positively by significant others in the social group, the child has a chance to blossom. A variety of social benefits have been identified for children with ADHD who are treated with the medication, including:

- Less controlling and critical behavior from parents.
- More positive and warmer interactions with parents.
- Fewer instances of being singled out by teachers.
- Better ratings by teachers.
- Less intense and controlling behavior from teachers.
- Better social reactions and responses from peers.
- More positive ratings by peers (e.g., more likely to be rated as "fun" or as "a best friend").
- Less aggression toward peers.
- Enhancement of social standing with peers.

In addition to providing educational and social benefits, medications may also affect the way that children see themselves. For example, some children suffer from years of failure before being prescribed effective medication. Medication can enhance associations between how children see themselves and how well they do on tasks (Milich, Licht, Murphy, & Pelham, 1989). Children benefit immensely from success experiences.

OPPORTUNITIES FOR CONTRIBUTIONS
FROM SCHOOL PERSONNEL

Psychotropic medications are only one component of comprehensive treatment programs for children and adolescents. They can often alleviate serious symptoms and so give a child a chance to benefit from other interventions, such as a special education classroom, social skills training, or a behavior management program. Until the child is on a level playing field with other children, the child's capabilities are not really known.

Many parents and professionals believe that physicians manage all issues related to medication. However, especially in the case of psychotropic medication, physicians are very much in need of information. The more information, the better the management of the child's problem. School personnel are privy to so much behavioral and emotional data that are valuable to physicians and pediatric psychologists in the evaluation of the efficacy and power of a child's treatment program. Physicians often rely heavily on feedback from parents and other people in the child's environment to make decisions about the best medications and whether or not changes are necessary in the child's treatment plan.

Most psychotropic medications are prescribed for conditions that cannot be diagnosed with a blood test or other laboratory measures. Instead, conditions like ADHD, depression, and obsessive–compulsive disorder are diagnosed by obtaining information from the child, the parent, and other adults in the child's life. Physicians often see children in their office for less than an hour before making a diagnosis and prescribing treatment. Information from people who interact with the child is invaluable toward the accuracy of diagnosis. Teacher and parent input are necessary and crucial in making positive treatment choices.

The following paragraphs describe some of the roles that school personnel may play in medication management for children.

Identifying Symptoms

School professionals are often in a unique position to provide information about a child's behavior. Problems that may be tolerable or overlooked at home may cause trouble at school (e.g., difficulty sitting still, difficulty concentrating). Similarly, many parents are not trained in the concepts of developmental norms. Developmental norms are the types of skills and behaviors a child should display at specific ages. School personnel, however, are well versed in the types of tasks a child would be expected to complete at particular grade levels. On a day-to-day basis, teachers can compare a child's skills and behaviors to those of the peer group and make better determinations about normal versus outside-the-norm behaviors. For example, kindergartners are sometimes shy with adults, but a teacher can usually separate normal shyness from a more significant problem like anxiety disorder or separation anxiety. Also, most parents and physicians do not have the extensive opportunity to observe the child during interactions with other children. Such information can prove to be essential in making certain diagnoses (e.g., autism spectrum disorders).

Providing Feedback on Treatment Efficacy

Psychotropic medication is often prescribed for behaviors or problems that are difficult to measure, and school personnel are often asked to provide feedback to parents and physicians on treatment efficacy. This is particularly important when the medication has been prescribed to improve the child's ability to learn, as in the case of stimulant treatment for ADHD. Teachers hold the golden key to a primary measure of success of the medication.

Another value of feedback from teachers is that children may lack the skills needed to communicate changes (both positive and negative) associated with psychotropic medications. Physicians often need information from teachers and other adults in the child's environment to assess medication response and side effects. Teachers, school nurses, and school administrators can be informed of medication changes and alert the primary care provider. In some cases, teachers can deliberately be kept blind to medication changes and so may be more objective in assessing changes in the child's behavior. In either situation, primary care providers may request weekly checklists from teachers during the initial phase of medication adjustment to find the best treatment for the child's difficulties.

Monitoring Adverse Side Effects

Medications can improve classroom behavior and these improvements can in turn result in improved academic performance. However, psychotropic medications are also sometimes associated with adverse side effects that can compromise behavior and learning. Some side effects, like minor fatigue or irritability, may be relatively benign. Other adverse side effects can be serious. An example is tardive dyskinesia, which is a syndrome of involuntary movements associated with long-term use of antipsychotic medications. When tardive dyskinesia is observed, swift action can prevent long-lasting damage. Some medications can also lower a child's seizure threshold, making seizures more likely. Other medications may induce tics. It is important that all adults in the child's environment are aware of the side effects associated with a child's medications. If adults who spend significant time with the medicated child know what to look for, physicians can be alerted quickly to a possible adverse reaction.

Ensuring Treatment Adherence

Some psychotropic medications must be taken several times a day, including during school hours. Some of these medications may be taken as needed—referred to as a PRN (*pro re nata*) or flexible schedule—and other medications must be taken at very specific times. Individuals working directly with the child must often track the times the child is expected to take medication. Additionally, as budget cutbacks reduce school nursing services, the responsibility for actually administering medications may fall on teachers, the school counselor, or even the school secretary. It is vital that individuals involved with providing medications be familiar with medication-specific factors. Depending on the medication, this information may include:

- The window of time during which the child must receive a medication.
- How to respond if a dose is missed.
- How to respond if a child accidentally takes two doses of the medication.
- Knowing if the child needs to be monitored to ensure the dose is actually taken and not cheeked and then thrown or given away.
- Whether the medication has the potential for abuse by others.

Promoting Positive Self-Image in Children Who Take Medications

Because medications are effective, they are being used more than ever for treatment of behavioral and emotional problems in children. Nonetheless, many families fear that their child will be stigmatized by taking medications. Family members may try to hide the fact that their child is taking medication. Children often notice this secrecy. Children who take medication for any condition (regardless of whether the condition is psychiatric in nature) are often very sensitive about this fact and are hesitant to tell their friends that they take medication or have a certain condition. In such cases, school personnel must be responsive to the child's awkwardness and desire for privacy. Further, if the child and family elect to do so, school personnel can help to educate classmates about the child's condition and the medication. This can go a long way toward reducing stigma and improving a child's self-image. The child who feels comfortable will probably be more likely to adhere to treatment.

MYTHS AND FACTS ABOUT CHILDREN AND MEDICATION

- *Myth:* Use of medication during childhood will result in increased risk of substance abuse during adolescence or adulthood.
- *Facts:* There is no evidence that children's early use of prescription medications to change feelings or behaviors will lead them to use illegal drugs when they are teenagers or adults. This issue has received a great deal of attention recently from researchers concerned with children with ADHD. Not only does medication management not lead to later substance abuse in this group of children, it actually protects children with ADHD against risk of later substance use (Faraone & Wilens, 2003; Fischer & Barkley, 2003). Biederman (2003) found that children with ADHD who were not treated with medications were three to four times more likely to have a substance use disorder during adolescence than children with ADHD who were treated with medications. Children who receive proper treatment may follow a more positive developmental track that will make them less likely to

abuse drugs or alcohol when they are older. Further, if the child has problems with impulsivity, as children with ADHD do, medication may make them less likely to make impulsive decisions to use drugs or alcohol.

- *Myth:* Medications make children act like "zombies."
- *Facts:* This is an area where teachers and other school personnel are especially important. Proper medication treatment should help children behave more normally and more like themselves. Most medications should not make the child appear blunted, sedated, or mentally foggy. If teachers observe such symptoms, they should alert physicians and parents so the child can be evaluated.

- *Myth:* If children are given medications, they will never learn to face their problems and will depend on medications to do it for them.
- *Facts:* For children with neurological abnormalities, using medication to normalize neurological functioning is similar to providing a hearing aid to a child with a hearing problem. We do not expect that a child with a hearing problem will learn to hear better if the hearing aid is withheld. Similarly, we do not expect a child with a neurological problem to improve without proper treatment. However, the definition of proper treatment varies from child to child and from disorder to disorder. Some disorders respond best to medication, some respond best to psychotherapy, and some respond best to a combination of therapy and medication. Again, the ongoing information provided by school personnel is indispensable to the primary treatment team as a coordinated treatment plan is implemented and monitored.

- *Myth:* A child may become addicted to the medication prescribed.
- *Facts:* Very few medications prescribed for learning and behavior in children have addictive properties as long as they are taken as prescribed. However, children who have been taking a medication regularly may show negative effects if the medication is withdrawn suddenly. Some medications must be tapered rather than abruptly discontinued. When it is time to discontinue medication, it is imperative that a physician supervise the tapering schedule.

- *Myth:* Medicated children need drug holidays.
- *Facts:* Some years ago, physicians and parents had concerns that stimulant medications such as methylphenidate (Ritalin) caused growth retardation. As a result, it was once popular to give children drug holidays (medication-free periods of time) to allow the child's growth to catch up to age norms. However, we now know that these medications do not affect children's height over the long term and that drug holidays are unnecessary. Planned drug holidays are appropriate when assessing further need for a particular medication in managing a specific problem. However, it is very important that parents consult with their physicians whenever they plan to withdraw a medication because withdrawing certain medications suddenly can be dangerous. For some severe behaviors and disorders, withdrawing treatment can place the child at risk for harm to self or others.

• *Myth:* Once the child finishes school, there will no longer be a need for medications for learning and behavior.

• *Facts:* Some children may require medication management for less than a year, but other children require long-term treatment. Many factors are entered into the decision-making algorithm for how long a child needs treatment. The primary considerations are the types and severity of the child's difficulties. Some problems may disappear without treatment, some are likely to abate with proper treatment, but treatable problems are unlikely to disappear completely. For example, children with depression are often treated with an antidepressant medication for a short period, say 6 months. However, if the child's depression recurs multiple times after medication is stopped, the physician may decide that medication needs to be maintained on a preventive basis over the long term. Similarly, some children with mild ADHD may only need to take medication on school days but not on weekends or during the summer. Children with more severe ADHD may need to take medication during college and adulthood.

• *Myth:* Medications will fix the child's behavior problems.

• *Facts:* It is extremely rare that a psychotropic medication will fix a child's difficulties entirely. The best treatment plans usually include a combination of appropriate educational interventions, therapy, and medications. For most children with emotional, learning, and behavior problems, medication may improve behavior, but other supports will continue to be necessary to help the child achieve success in school. In some cases, medication allows a child to benefit from an educational intervention. For example, a child with severe ADHD and a learning disability may be better able to retain information when taking medication. Similarly, a child with severe depression may respond better to psychotherapy when the depression is partially alleviated by medication.

HOW MEDICATIONS WORK

Pharmacology is the study of physical and chemical effects of drugs in the body, the ways in which these drugs work, and the effects these drugs have on body chemistry, physiology, and behavior. Psychopharmacology is the study of the effects of drugs on psychological processes and behavior. Behavioral psychopharmacology is the study of behavioral and cognitive response to psychotropic medication, or drugs that act on the mind. Pediatric psychopharmacology refers to the specific study of the effects of medications on the behavior of children. Pediatric psychopharmacology is different from adult psychopharmacology because children differ physiologically and psychologically from adults. For example, medications can be absorbed and metabolized differently by children.

Drugs or medications are chemical substances that affect the body. Medications are sometimes referred to as agents, which means that they are chemically active substances. Psychotropic agents are prescribed to alter mood or behavior. Medications are usually given at least two names, a generic name and a trade name. This practice can be confusing.

The generic name usually describes the medication's chemical formulation. The trade name is chosen by a pharmaceutical company to promote the medication. The trade name is usually shorter and easier to remember than the generic version and sometimes describes its therapeutic action. For example, Ritalin is a trade name for a medication for ADHD. The generic name for Ritalin is methylphenidate. One generic medication may have several trade names. In these cases, the chemical formulation of the drug is usually the same, but dosages or delivery systems vary. Because there is only one generic name for a specific medication but there may be several trade names, it is often easier to use the generic name. We primarily use generic names in this book. Appendix 1 lists the generic and trade names of mental health medications for children and gives a brief description of their use and side effects.

Some medications are available in regular drug stores or grocery stores without a prescription and are known as over-the-counter medications. Medications prescribed by a physician are called prescription medications. Access to prescription medications is controlled by physicians and pharmacists.

Some prescription medications are more likely to be abused than others. With some medications there is a risk that the substance will be diverted to someone besides the intended patient or will be used in a manner other than its legitimate medical use. Medications that are more easily misused are usually classified as controlled substances. Certain medications for pain management (e.g., opioid analgesics) and for management of symptoms of ADHD (e.g., methylphenidate) are controlled substances. Physicians and pharmacies must follow stricter regulations when providing controlled substances than when providing regular prescriptions because of the potential for abuse, addiction, and other problems. For example, physicians and pharmacists keep careful inventories of these medications.

Companies that manufacture medications are required to specify potential side effects and identify patients for whom a medication has been approved by the federal Food and Drug Administration (FDA). Very few psychotropic medications have been approved for use with children. Medications that are prescribed to children but not approved for children are being prescribed "off-label." Off-label means that the medication has been prescribed to a person or for a problem other than that for which it was originally researched and intended. For example, most stimulant medications are FDA-approved for children over 6 years old. However, stimulant treatments are often prescribed to children under the age of 6, even though the FDA has not specifically approved use with this population. Similarly, Prozac is the only antidepressant medication that is approved for use in the treatment of depression in children, but a variety of other antidepressants are also used.

A medication that has been approved for use with children for one problem (e.g., social anxiety disorder) may not be approved for use with children for another problem (e.g., obsessive–compulsive disorder). Medications are often used off-label with children and adults, mostly because studies have not been conducted with a specific population or a specific problem but have proved effective in other patients. Using a medication for an off-label use does not mean the medication is necessarily contraindicated for that use, is unsafe, or does not work. In many cases, studies that would get the medication approved by the FDA for the off-label use may not have been conducted because the risks may be too great for the target population (e.g., very young children) or because the problem is not sufficiently common (e.g., self-injurious behavior).

Administering Medication

Medications can be taken by several different methods, called routes. The method of administration can affect the speed at which the drug begins to act and the duration of its effect. See Table 1.1 for a summary of five common routes of medication administration. It is important that medications be taken in the manner in which they are prescribed because the physician makes a decision on the route based on the symptoms. A physician also needs to be consulted before any changes are made in the way a medication is taken. For example, some capsule medications are designed to allow the capsules to be opened up and poured into a drink or into soft food for easier consumption by children. Other capsules, such as time-release capsules, are not designed to be used in this manner.

Most psychotropic agents are administered orally as a pill or capsule. These medications are dissolved in the stomach and are absorbed through the walls of the digestive tract. The medication may be absorbed more quickly or more slowly depending on such factors as whether the child has a full stomach, is ill, or is taking other medications.

Monitoring Dosage

Some medications stay in the body for only a short time and others may remain in the body for longer periods. The half-life of a drug is the amount of time it takes for the body to reduce the amount of the drug by about 50%. Some medications, such as Prozac, have variable half-lives, and their effects may not be noticeable until the child has been taking the medication for several weeks. This process of building up levels of a medication is called accumulation. When accumulation is a factor, it can be difficult to determine whether behavioral changes are the effect of medication or other factors. Conversely, medications like Ritalin act very quickly and effects can be seen within an hour of administration. These medications may also exit the child's system more quickly than medications that must accumulate.

TABLE 1.1. Routes of Medication Administration

Route of administration	Benefits
Oral (swallowed)	Convenient, but absorption rates may vary.
Sublingual (under the tongue)	Convenient and quickly absorbed.
Rectal (inserted into the anus)	Helpful for nausea and vomiting.
Inhalation	Medication enters bloodstream rapidly through lungs.
Injection	Medication enters bloodstream rapidly.

Before making medications available to the public, companies that manufacture them must conduct careful studies to determine the effects of various doses. For the individual, however, finding the correct dose can be complicated. Very low doses of medications often do not produce the desired effects, but very high doses may be harmful. When a child starts a new medication, it is usually a small dose. The physician may then adjust the dose until the desired effect is achieved or until adverse effects are observed. This process of adjusting the dose of a medication is called titration. Most psychotropic medications prescribed for managing learning and behavior problems in children must be carefully titrated to determine a dose that is most effective and does not cause adverse effects. When adverse effects are observed, the physician may decrease the dose, change the medication, or prescribe a second medication to control the adverse effects of the first. Because there are often striking individual differences in drug response, it may take some time before optimal medication and dosage are found. Further, because children are still growing physically, changes in weight and body chemistry may also change medication efficacy, and medications may need to be changed over time.

Addiction, Tolerance, and Withdrawal

Addiction is a pattern of drug use that is characterized by compulsive and harmful use of a drug and the tendency to relapse when the drug is withdrawn. Many people are concerned about the possibility of drug addiction. A medication that has been prescribed for a legitimate medical use can be abused as easily as street drugs. Addiction as a term has been applied widely in our culture. Substance abuse is a maladaptive pattern of substance use that leads to impairment in life functions, such as failing school, having legal problems, driving while intoxicated, and having interpersonal problems (American Psychiatric Association, 2000).

A more serious pattern of behavior is known as substance dependence. In substance dependence, the person continues to take the drug despite serious, sometimes life-threatening, drug-related problems. In some cases, the person may show signs of physiological dependence, such as tolerance or withdrawal. Tolerance occurs when a dose that previously had an effect on the individual no longer produces the desired effect. The individual must take more of the medication to produce the same effect. As a practical and familiar example, some adults who drink a cup of coffee in the morning to wake up find that they need more coffee to experience the wake-up effect. Tolerance may be behavioral (when the individual counteracts the behavioral effects of the drug) or metabolic (when the individual's body counteracts drug effects through metabolic processes). Withdrawal symptoms occur when a person stops taking a medication. For example, a regular coffee drinker who does not have a morning cup of coffee may experience headache or fatigue.

Sometimes drug dependence is experienced even when the medication has not been abused. Some children on stimulant drug therapy for ADHD may show increased inattentiveness and overactivity from baseline levels when the drug wears off. This is known as the rebound phenomenon. When this occurs, the child's physician should be alerted so that a medication change can be considered. A baseline level is the intensity or number of symptoms a child had before medications were prescribed.

Interactions and Adverse Effects

Children are often prescribed more than one medication to manage a constellation of behavioral, learning, and health problems. Many children with chronic health problems like seizure disorders, sickle cell disease, or diabetes receive medication to treat their health problems as well as medication for learning and behavior. Multiple medications may be prescribed to manage multiple disorders (polypharmacy) or to treat the same disorder (multiple drug therapy). Interactions can occur when one drug affects the other by increasing toxicity or decreasing efficacy. Physicians who treat children with multiple conditions must be especially vigilant when choosing medications so harmful interactions are avoided. In fact, many pharmacies have computers with programs that alert the druggist to harmful interactions between medications.

Ideally, a medication would treat only the child's symptom and would not affect any other parts of the child's physical or social life. Unfortunately, most medications that treat learning and behavior disorders produce undesired effects. Adverse effects (side effects) are unwanted physiological, behavioral, or cognitive effects that are associated with medications. In some cases, the adverse effect may be related to dose. An optimal dose of a stimulant treatment for ADHD may decrease hyperactivity and impulsivity while an excessive dose might make the child appear overly passive, quiet, and out of sync with the environment. Behavioral or cognitive toxicity occurs when a medication prevents an adaptive behavior from occurring or impairs cognitive functioning. Certain antipsychotic medications, for example, may sedate the child and make social interactions with peers more difficult. Certain medications prescribed for seizure management may cause the child to have difficulty with information processing, which can impair school performance.

The Central Nervous System

Scientists now have a good understanding of how the brain works and the origins of learning and emotional problems. In some cases, these problems can be traced to specific abnormalities in brain function, and medications can be prescribed to help the child's brain function more normally. Medications prescribed for learning and behavior problems usually affect the central nervous system (CNS). The CNS consists of the brain and spinal cord. The CNS is made of cells called neurons (Figure 1.1) that conduct information between parts of the brain and between the body and the brain. The neuron's cell body is called the soma. The most common pathway for neurons to send information from the soma to other neurons is through long, slender branches that project off the soma. These projections are called axons. Neurons also receive information into the soma from other neurons through branches (dendrites) that extend from the soma. Different types of neurons conduct different types of information. Motor neurons send information to the muscles of the body to make the body move in a desired way. Sensory neurons conduct information from the outside world (vision, touch, smell) to parts of the brain so that this information can be processed. Interneurons send information from one part of the brain to another.

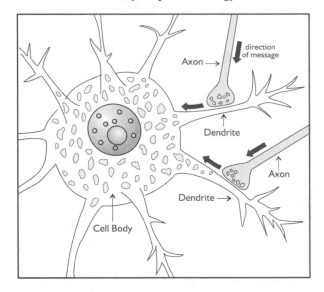

FIGURE 1.1. Neuron (nerve cell). From *The Anatomy Coloring Book*, 3rd ed., by Wynn Kapit and Lawrence M. Elson. Copyright 2002 by Wynn Kapit and Lawrence M. Elson. Reprinted by permission of Pearson Education, Inc.

Neurons "talk" to each other by sending chemical signals. The chemicals used to send these messages are called neurotransmitters. There are many different types of neurotransmitter chemicals that have different purposes and act in different parts of the brain. Table 1.2 describes the five major types of neurotransmitters that affect learning and behavior. Acetylcholine (ACH) is found in the brain and spinal cord. It helps communicate information about movement and is important in learning, memory, and sleep. Catecholamines are a class of neurotransmitters that include norepinephrine, epinephrine, and dopamine (see Table 1.3). Catecholamines are very important in the regulation of mood and behavior.

TABLE 1.2. Types of Neurotransmitters

Neurotransmitter	Function	Associated problems
Acetylcholine	Excitatory neurotransmitter that mediates neuromuscular transmission and parasympathetic arousal.	Alzheimer's disease
Catecholamines	Involved in personality, mood, and drive states.	Schizophrenia, mood disorders
Serotonin	Suppression of arousal, regulation of hunger and temperature, sexual behavior, aggression, and sleep onset.	Mood and anxiety disorders
GABA (gamma-aminobutyric acid)	Inhibits behavior.	Anxiety disorders
Endorphins	Inhibit pain.	Addiction

TABLE 1.3. Types of Catecholamines

Type of Catecholamine	Associated problems
Norepinephrine	Mania, depression, ADHD
Epinephrine	Anxiety
Dopamine	Schizophrenia, depression

Serotonin is a neurotransmitter that is important in the regulation of mood, appetite, arousal, and aggression. Many popular antidepressants target serotonergic activity. GABA (gamma-aminobutyric acid) is a neurotransmitter that inhibits the activity of neurons. A person who does not have enough GABA may become anxious or may show excess movement. Endorphins are important in inhibiting pain. When a person is hurt, endorphins are immediately released in the brain to limit pain.

Neurons release neurotransmitters from their axons to send signals to the dendrites of other neurons in order to communicate information. The space or cleft between one neuron and its neighboring neurons is known as a synapse (Figure 1.2). If a neuron releases too much of a neurotransmitter into a synapse, that neuron can reabsorb the neurotransmitter. This process of taking a released neurotransmitter substance back into the cell is known as reuptake. Neurons "read" the chemical signals being sent out from the axons of their neighbors. Once a sufficient level of the right kind of chemical (neurotransmitter) has been detected, a neuron will fire, or send, its own message. In other words, it will send out its own chemical signal to other neurons down the message path by releasing its own neurotransmitters.

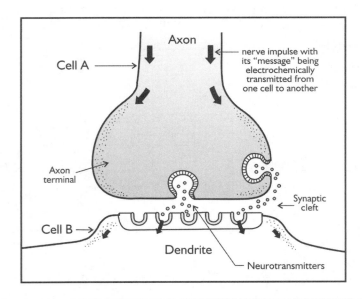

FIGURE 1.2. Synapse. From *The Anatomy Coloring Book*, 3rd ed., by Wynn Kapit and Lawrence M. Elson. Copyright 2002 by Wynn Kapit and Lawrence M. Elson. Reprinted by permission of Pearson Education, Inc.

When neurons release too much or too little of a neurotransmitter, problems can develop that can affect the way the person feels or behaves. Most medications prescribed to help children with behavioral or emotional problems affect specific neurotransmitters in the brain. There are several ways these medications can work. They may cause neurons to produce more or less of a neurotransmitter, they may cause the neurons to release more or less of a neurotransmitter into the synaptic cleft, they may make the neuron more or less likely to reabsorb a neurotransmitter that has already been released (reuptake), or they may make other neurons more or less sensitive to the effects of the neurotransmitter.

SUMMARY

Over the past 50 years, our understanding of how the brain develops and works and of the problems that can result when brain function or development is abnormal have advanced dramatically. We also now have access to vastly improved techniques for early identification of children who have emotional, learning, and behavior problems. We have a new and improved arsenal of treatments to help these at-risk children be successful in their home, school, and social environments. One result of these advances in understanding, identification, and treatment is that more school-age children are likely to be prescribed medication for a wider variety of problems than before. Each of these children has unique needs related to a treatment regimen.

It is becoming essential from treatment and ethical standpoints that professionals working with children in schools have an understanding of childhood disorders and the medications used to manage these disorders. This book provides an overview of medications, disorders, and medication-related issues for educators who work with children who have emotional, behavioral, and learning problems. We illustrate concepts through the use of case studies. Reproducible checklists, data sheets, and tables are provided.

Although each child's needs are different, we aim to provide practical information that can be applied to a broad range of children who are served by the educational system. Children with developmental delays, emotional difficulties, learning problems, behavior problems, and other childhood disorders will profit from the knowledge gained by teachers who have garnered information from this book.

REFERENCES

Aman, M. G., Van Bourgondien, M. E., Wolford, P. L., & Sarphare, G. (1995). Psychotropic and anticonvulsant drugs in subjects with autism: Prevalence and patterns of use. *Journal of the American Academy of Child and Adolescent Psychiatry, 34*, 1672–1681.

American Psychiatric Association. (2000). *Diagnostic and statistical manual of mental disorders* (4th ed., text rev.). Washington, DC: Author.

Biederman, J. (2003). Pharmacotherapy for attention-deficit/hyperactivity disorder (ADHD) decreases the risk for substance abuse: Findings from a longitudinal follow-up of youths with and without ADHD. *Journal of Clinical Psychiatry, 64*(Suppl. 11), 3–8.

Emslie, G. J., Mayes, T. L., & Hughes, C. W. (2000). Update in the pharmacological treatment of childhood depression. *Psychiatric Clinics of North America, 23,* 811–821.

Faraone, S. V., & Wilens, T. (2003). Does stimulant treatment lead to substance use disorders? *Journal of Clinical Psychiatry, 64*(Suppl. 11), 9–13.

Fischer, M., & Barkley, R. A. (2003). Childhood stimulant treatment and risk for later substance abuse. *Journal of Clinical Psychiatry, 64*(Suppl. 11), 19–23.

Fox, M. H., Foster, C. H., & Zito, J. M. (2000). Building pharmacoepidemiological capacity to monitor psychotropic drug use among children enrolled in Medicaid. *American Journal of Medical Quality, 15*(4), 126–136.

Gadow, K. D. (1993). Prevalence of drug therapy. In J. S. Werry & M. G. Aman (Eds.), *Practitioner's guide to psychoactive drugs for children and adolescents* (pp. 57–74). New York: Plenum Press.

Milich, R., Licht, B. G., Murphy, D. A., & Pelham, W. E. (1989). Attention-deficit/ hyperactivity disordered boys' evaluations of and attributions for task performance on medication versus placebo. *Journal of Abnormal Psychology, 98*(3), 280–284.

Perl, R. (1992, November 8). Overdosing on Ritalin. *The Atlanta Journal Constitution,* pp. 7–9.

Safer, D. J., & Krager, J. M. (1988). A survey of medication treatment for hyperactive/inattentive students. *Journal of the American Medical Association, 260,* 2256–2258.

Safer, D. J., Zito, J. M., & Fine, E. M. (1996). Increased methylphenidate usage for attention deficit disorder in the 1990s [see comment]. *Pediatrics, 98,* 1084–1088.

Vitiello, B. (2001). Psychopharmacology for young children: Clinical needs and research opportunities. *Pediatrics, 108,* 983–989.

2

The Importance of School Personnel on the Treatment Team

The rapid increase in use of psychotropic medications with children has created practical, legal, and ethical concerns for schools. In Chapter 1, you learned about effective treatments for many disorders. This chapter provides tools to track the effects of medication and guidelines for talking to parents to resolve behavior or treatment problems. Finding the appropriate time and way to talk to a family can be difficult. Teachers may harbor reasonable frustration when they are not consulted about a child's behaviors or when they are not informed about changes in a child's treatment plan. The actual provision of psychotropic medications by the school can be especially problematic because of legal issues involving consent, safety, and liability. Even the most effective treatments are subject to failure if the child or family does not fully support the treatment choice. School personnel are often in a position to counsel and encourage the child and family toward treatment adherence.

In this chapter, we address the unique issues of psychotropic medications prescribed for children. We present effective strategies for communicating with parents, physicians, and other mental health professionals, and we provide an overview of the referral process for a child whose behavior may indicate a disorder or disability. Practical issues of children taking medications at school, legal questions, and attitudes toward treatment acceptability are discussed.

COMMUNICATING WITH PARENTS

One of the most challenging issues that teachers face in managing students with learning and behavior problems is deciding when and how to talk to parents about these concerns. Often, teachers are concerned about appearing overly negative about a child. In other cases, they are hesitant to bring up concerns because they are not absolutely sure a problem exists. Some teachers are afraid they will be considered responsible for not being able to manage a child's behavior better. The most important rule to remember is that, as a professional charged with the education of a child, you must let the child's parent know if you think something is getting in the way of the child receiving an appropriate education. Your choice is not about whether to discuss your concerns with parents but when and how to talk about these concerns. More than likely, the parents have already noticed the problem. The following "dos" and "don'ts" will help you effectively communicate to parents your concerns about a child's learning and behavior.

Don't Suggest That the Child Needs Medication

Only a physician can determine whether a child might benefit from medication. Instead of making specific treatment recommendations, it is more helpful to tell the child's parents exactly what your concerns are, especially with examples of the child's behavior. Then it makes sense for you to suggest that they talk about these concerns with their child's physician. Families need hope that things can get better, and letting them know that a health care provider can offer treatments will add to their hope.

　　If a child is having a problem, there are usually several treatment options. Here is a sample conversation you might have with a child's father:

> "Mr. Robbins, Matthew seems to be having a very hard time staying in his chair during work times. He runs around the room and misses a lot of instruction because he can't seem to stay in his chair and pay attention. Keeping still is a lot more challenging for him than for the other kids in class. I've also noticed that the other children have a hard time playing with him because he is always on the go and can't seem to settle down to concentrate on a particular game. He may be missing out on some friendships because of this. Is this something that you have noticed at home or when you take him places like baseball games or movies? It might be helpful to talk to his pediatrician about these concerns. If his physician decides that Matthew does have a problem, there are a lot of different treatment options that might make school and friendships easier for him."

Do Be as Specific as Possible When Communicating Concerns

Try not to rely on labels like "he's hyperactive," "she's acting out," or "he's depressed." These words are vague and can mean different things to different people.

　　It can be helpful to keep a log of observations for one week before meeting with a family so that specific examples can be shared:

> November 1, 11:22 . Told class to put their art away and to take out their reading. Alyssa started to cry and said she wanted to finish. Let her know she could finish later. She tore

up the picture and threw it. She started to cry and scream, "I hate you" and "I'm going to kill all of you." She cried for about 20 minutes.

Appendix 2 can be used to keep track of these observations. This form should only be used as a starting point for communicating concerns to the child's parents. It is usually not necessary or helpful to keep this type of observation form for more than a week, unless the behavior of concern happens only rarely. In later phases of assessment and treatment, other types of forms that collect more or different information (e.g., antecedent–behavior–consequence) are usually more appropriate. If you need to use shorthand and abbreviations to take notes, take a few minutes at the end of each day to expand the notes so that they can be understood by others. Record only observations that can be seen or heard and not your interpretations of the situation. Record the duration of the behavior. Figure 2.1 is an example of a completed Event Observation Log. In this case, Lilliana's teacher, Ms. Duff, is concerned about Lilliana's anxiety level. Lilliana has missed 10 days of school since the beginning of the year, and all of her absences have occurred on test days. She also talks excessively about exams and seems to suffer from constant headaches and stomachaches. To make this information especially useful to the family and physician, Ms. Duff can attach a copy of Lilliana's nurse-visit record and attendance record to this form. Lilliana's parents can share this form with Lilliana's physician.

Don't Minimize Your Concerns

Be honest with the child's parents about the behaviors that are interfering with the child's living and learning. If you think a problem exists, the child's family needs to know. Many teachers are afraid of alarming parents unnecessarily. It is far better to correct a problem than to allow a child who needs help to go months or years without receiving it. Usually, the earlier a problem is identified, the easier it is to treat. For example, some children with inattentive-type ADHD may not be diagnosed until fifth or sixth grade. By the time the problem is identified, these children may have fallen far behind in school, may have lost self-confidence, and may believe that they will never catch up. Professionals who are afraid of upsetting parents by telling them their concerns (or by minimizing concerns) are not helping the child or the family, and serious consequences may occur. Years later, the family may wonder why no one told them that their child was struggling.

Do Remember That Your Opinion Is Important

If you suspect that there is something different about a child, let that child's family know exactly what your concerns are. Some school personnel are reluctant to talk to parents about concerns because their knowledge of specific disorders is limited. It is important to remember that you are a professional who knows about children, even if you don't know exactly how to diagnose their problems. Many parents do not have expertise in child development and don't have the opportunity to see how other children behave and function. Remember that your opinion, knowledge, and observations are valuable.

Event Observation Log

Child's name: *Lilliana*   Teacher's name: *Ms. Duff*

Week of: *10/09*

Date	Time	Event
10/9	8:30	L forgot her lunch money and worried that she would not have lunch. Told her the cafeteria would give her lunch. She continued to worry for the next three hours that she would not get lunch.
10/9	1:15	Told the class there would be a pop quiz in history. Halfway through the test, L asked to go to the nurse due to a stomachache.
10/10	3:00	Today was L's day to be student of the day and she did not come to school. Same thing happened last time she was to be student of the day.
10/11	9:45	L is asking an excessive number of questions about Friday's big science exam. She was told not to ask about the exam again, but she continued to ask. I told her that if she asked again, the consequence would be one docked grade.
10/11	10:20	L asked to go to the nurse due to a stomachache.
10/12	11:00	L is complaining of a headache.
10/12	1:30	L continues to worry about tomorrow's exam. I let her know that if she misses the exam, the consequence will be an essay make-up test.
10/12	2:20	L continues to complain of headache from this morning.
10/13	7:30	L's mother called to say she was throwing up this morning and will not be at school. Thus, she missed the exam.

FIGURE 2.1. Example of completed Event Observation Log.

Don't Suggest a Specific Medication

There may be times when you are almost certain that a medication is not helping a child and that another medication might work better. However, only a health care provider with expertise in pediatric disorders should make recommendations or decisions about what types of medications (if any) a child might need. Not only is it inappropriate for nonmedical personnel to make medication recommendations, but this type of behavior can make the school district vulnerable to lawsuits if the child experiences an adverse reaction to a medication. Avoid statements like "I had another child with similar problems as Michelle who did great after he started taking (Risperdal, Celexa, Ritalin, etc.). Maybe you should try that." Instead, make a statement such as "I know there are many different ways that physicians can help children with these problems. Why don't you talk to your child's physician and see what treatment options are suggested?" At the same time, you can offer to provide the child's physician with data about the child's behavior.

Do Offer to Send a Letter to the Child's Physician

Appendix 3 outlines a letter you can complete for parents to give to their child's physician. An example of a completed physician letter can be found in Figure 2.2. In the example, the child's teacher had concerns about poor reading comprehension, obsessive behaviors, and poor social skills. Her letter provided information to help the physician arrive at the best treatment. Be as specific as possible about your concerns and provide the physician with a variety of examples. For instance, instead of saying that a child is rude, give several examples of rude behavior so the physician knows whether you mean the child is naive to social rules or is oppositional. It may also be helpful to complete the checklist in Appendix 4 and attach it to the letter. This form is used to note problems you observed in the child and to rate problems that are of greatest concern. For example, you might note that a child is distractible, but the form also allows you to let the family and physician know you are more concerned about aggression. Distractibility is less of a concern even though it is a problem. Attaching a copy of the observations you shared with the child's parents (see Appendix 2) may also be helpful. Finally, consider attaching one or two examples of the child's work and report cards.

Don't Wait to Contact Parents if Serious Behavior Problems Are Observed

In many cases, it makes sense to take a few days to gather information to share with parents before meeting with them. This will ensure that parents understand exactly what you saw in their child, what your concerns are, and how serious they are. However, there are some danger signs that necessitate immediate parental contact. These signs are too serious to take time to collect further information. If any of these behaviors are seen or suspected, school administrators should be notified and parents contacted the same day. These danger signs include:

As _Jaylen_ 's teacher, I have been asked to provide the following information about school-related issues and progress.

Child's name: _Jaylen Carter_   Child's grade: _3_

Form completed by: _Jill Rover_   Position: _Teacher_

Type of classroom: _Regular Education_   School: _Oakbrook_

Telephone: _555-0403_   Best times to call: _7:30 A.M._

This child's academic difficulties include:

Reading comprehension is very poor. He can read an entire story, yet be unable to answer simple questions about it.

This child's academic strengths include:

Excellent decoding skills. Does great in math except on word problems. Does better with rote skills such as memorizing spelling words.

This child's behavioral difficulties include:

Meltdowns (crying, refusing to work, trying to leave the classroom) when things don't go his way (especially when he doesn't earn his stars, our behavior system). He has at least one meltdown a day and cries for 10 to 20 minutes each time. Even when he is not having a meltdown, his facial expression is almost always angry. He is constantly irritable.

This child's behavioral strengths include:

He tries very hard to earn his stars each day. He seems to want to behave better. He knows a lot about bugs!

Does this child have friends? Describe any social difficulties or problems.

No. The other children avoid him because he gets upset so easily. He also does not know what to say to other kids. He spends recess time scavenging for bugs.

Describe any unusual behaviors.

He talks about bugs to the exclusion of most other topics.

Is this child absent often? YES (NO) If yes, for what reason(s)?

(Jaylen is preoccupied with earning stars. He would come to school sick rather than miss stars.)

Questions/concerns about this child.

How can we prevent his meltdowns? How can we make him laugh and smile? How can we improve reading comprehension? How can we increase his chances for friendships?

Attach work sample, report card, and behavior observations to this form.

FIGURE 2.2. Example of letter to physician.

- Talking about death or suicide.
- Harming others or threatening to harm others.
- Seeing or hearing things that are not there.
- Self-harm (cutting arms, banging head) or talking about self-harm.
- Suspected substance abuse.

Treat these problems similarly to the way you would treat serious physical problems.

Do Communicate Your Concerns Empathically

This seems obvious but bears saying. Parents need to know that school personnel care about the child and the family and that you have the child's best interests in mind. Many parents think they may be blamed for the child's problems. Be sure to let parents know that children have difficulties for all kinds of reasons and that their child's physician can help them figure out why their child is struggling. The first person to tell parents that their child may have a problem may receive an angry or ambivalent response. Put yourself in their shoes as they try to grasp this information. Their response can often be calmed by consistently letting the family know that you are communicating out of concern for the child and that you believe the school, family, and physician, working together, may be able to do more to help the child succeed.

COMMUNICATING WITH PHYSICIANS AND OTHER MENTAL HEALTH PROFESSIONALS

Before talking with any physician or professional outside the school, be sure that you have consulted with your school administrators and are following school policy. Also, make sure the appropriate consent forms have been signed by the child's parent or legal guardian. If someone from a health center contacts you about a child, inform that person that you will require a signed release form from the parents before you can talk about the child. Ideally, the school administrator's or physician's office should have the parent sign an official consent form. In some emergency cases, verbal consent can be documented, but this is not ideal. In this era of fax machines and overnight deliveries, it is almost always possible to obtain an official written consent before talking to professionals outside the school. Usually it is not necessary to obtain consent to talk to other professionals employed in your school district. Once the consent form has been obtained, review it to determine if it is a one-way or two-way consent. One-way consent allows the school to provide information to the physician but does not allow the physician to provide information to the school, or vice versa. Two-way consent allows for an exchange of information between both parties. Two-way consent is ideal because it allows the school to ask the physician questions about the child's diagnosis and treatment plan.

Once parental consent has been documented, the school is free to provide information delineated on the form to the health care professional. We recommend that all contact with professionals outside the school be carefully documented. If a checklist or other form is completed, make a copy of it, date it, and place it in the child's file. If a telephone contact is made, take notes while you are talking, use these notes or write a summary of the conversation, sign and date this information, and place it in the child's file. This documentation process serves two purposes. First, if the forms are lost or cannot be located, this information will be available and won't need to be redone. Second, some children may be referred to multiple professionals before an accurate diagnosis is made, and each professional may ask the child's teacher for checklists and other information. If copies have been made, the teacher may not have to fill out a new form each time the child sees another provider. Third, if parents ask what was said about their child, this information will be easily available. In the worst circumstance, if a lawsuit is levied against the school district, this type of documentation can make the difference between a quick resolution and a lengthy legal dispute.

Some physicians will ask the school to complete a specific checklist or form about the child. Others may be interested in a phone conversation about the child's general behavior and academic performance. In either case, offer to fax or mail your Event Observation Log (Appendix 2), your letter to the child's physician (Appendix 3), or your Behavior Observation Form (Appendix 11, discussed in Chapter 5) to the professional. Before talking to the physician, it can also be helpful to go through the Problem Behavior Ranking Form (Appendix 4). As in communication with parents, do not minimize or exaggerate a child's problems. This will not help the child and can result in the development of an inappropriate and ineffective treatment plan.

Remember to think carefully about what information you want to share with professionals outside the school and how you will present that information. It can be difficult to identify the line between sharing relevant information with the physician (e.g., this child often comes to school smelling of urine) versus sharing information that is not relevant to the child's care (e.g., the child's mother has been divorced four times). It can be helpful to ask yourself whether you would be upset if the physician shared the information you provided with the family. If the answer is yes, it may still be appropriate to share the information, but you should do so in a way that is objective and professional. For example, rather than saying "I think her mom is too busy with her own life to take adequate care of Maggie" say, "I am concerned that Maggie often comes to school with unwashed hair and smelling of urine." The second example is an objective observation that does not cast blame on the family and is one that could be shared directly with the family.

THE REFERRAL PROCESS

Many school professionals wonder what happens once they have expressed concern to a child's parent. In most cases, the parent will contact the child's primary care physician, who will have a professional in the office conduct a screening evaluation. This brief evaluation provides information to determine if the child is at risk for developmental, learning, or behavior problems. If the screener indicates a problem, the physician will either conduct an in-depth evaluation or refer the child to a specialist. For example, in the case of ADHD, some primary care physicians are comfortable diagnosing and treating the disorder themselves, but others refer the child to a professional who specializes in ADHD. In the case of very complicated or more rare disorders such as autism or pediatric bipolar disorder, most primary care physicians will refer children to a specialist. Often, the specialist is a child psychiatrist or psychologist.

Depending on the nature of the child's difficulties, a diagnostic evaluation may be as short as an hour or as long as 2 or 3 days. In most cases, the professional will interview the parents and observe the child. A developmental, medical, educational, and social history will usually be obtained. Older children are often interviewed directly as well. When appropriate, physical tests like blood draws and brain scans may be conducted to rule out physical causes for the child's difficulties. Other tests, such as parent and teacher checklists and direct assessments of the child, may also be conducted. After the child has been evaluated, the physician will explain the child's diagnosis to the parents and offer one or more treatment or management options. Some physicians will actually provide treatment themselves. Specialists may refer the child back to the pediatrician or another health care provider to receive treatment once a diagnosis has been made and a treatment plan has been agreed upon.

There are many types of physicians who assess and treat children with behavioral, developmental, and emotional problems:

- A *pediatrician* is a medical doctor who specializes in child health care. Pediatricians conduct physicals and vaccinations and provide general medical care. Pediatricians often serve as gatekeepers to treatment by deciding when children need to be referred to other child specialists.
- A *pediatric neurologist* is a physician who specializes in diagnosing and treating problems in the brain, spinal cord, muscles, and nervous system. Pediatric neurologists often provide care for children who have a seizure disorder or who have suffered head injuries or strokes.
- A *child psychiatrist* is a medical doctor with expertise in diagnosing and treating psychiatric disorders in children. Child psychiatrists have expertise in the use of medications for psychiatric disorders in children. Some psychiatrists also provide counseling or other nonmedication therapy services.
- A *developmental pediatrician* is a pediatrician with expertise in the assessment and clinical management of children with disabilities. They have completed specialty training in developmental and behavioral pediatrics or neurodevelopmental disabilities. They will often prescribe and monitor medications for children with disabilities.
- A *pediatric or child clinical psychologist* has a doctorate but is not a medical doctor. However, these professionals receive intensive training in childhood psychiatric disorders. They specialize in the assessment and treatment of developmental, learning, behavioral, and psychiatric problems in children. Although most psychologists cannot prescribe medication, they often provide psychosocial interventions (e.g., parent training, therapy) for children with disabilities and other psychiatric disor-

ders. Several states and the military allow psychologists to prescribe psychotropic medications after receiving specialized training.

- A *school psychologist* may have a master's degree or a doctorate. School psychologists have specialized training in psychology and education. They provide assessment and intervention for school-age children with developmental, learning, and behavior problems. They do not prescribe medications. They may provide psychosocial interventions similar to those by pediatric psychologists.

ADMINISTERING MEDICATION AT SCHOOL

All school personnel should be aware of general issues relating to medication for children whether they administer the medication or not. Appendix 5 outlines general principles about medication and can be provided to all school employees. All school personnel (including bus drivers, gym teachers, therapists, and others) should be aware of this general information.

When a parent alerts the school that a child will be starting or changing medications, the parent should be asked to provide information about the medication. Parents can complete a Medication Initiation Form (Appendix 6) and then review it with school officials. Information from the form will provide school personnel with information about the medication and its side effects. The child's parents are also asked to decide how problem situations should be handled. It may seem unprofessional to ask a parent how the school should handle mistakes like a late dose or a missed dose of medication. In a perfect world, such mistakes would never happen. However, in the real world, mistakes do happen and it is essential that the school be prepared to handle problems when they arise. Some medications should be taken as soon as they are remembered and others may require that a dose be skipped if the medication is late. For some medications, an occasional missed dose may not be especially problematic; but, for others, a missed dose can result in serious problems. These specifics vary depending on the medication and the child.

Three types of forms may be necessary whenever a child is prescribed a new medication.

Medication Initiation Form

Parents should complete this or a similar form (Appendix 6) even when medications will not be directly provided at school. Children spend half of their waking hours at school, so school officials need to have information about possible side effects and potentially dangerous reactions associated with the medication the child is taking. Help can then be provided appropriately and an urgent problem will be recognized. In addition, the child's teachers will need to know basic information about the child's medications. For example, a teacher might need to know what to do when a child forgets to take medications before coming to school that morning.

Authorization to Administer Medication

Before any medication is administered at school, the child's parent and physician should be asked to provide a written statement that includes the name of the medication, the dose, the time the medication is to be taken, and the reason the medication has been prescribed. We suggest that the family be asked to complete a consent form to authorize the administration of medication. Many school districts have their own consent forms. If one is not available in your district, the form in Appendix 7 can be used.

Medication Log

The two primary purposes for the medication log are to track medication that has been provided to the school and to keep a record of the times the medication was given to the child. When filled out accurately, it provides documentation of what happened to each pill that the school received. This discourages theft of medication. Some schools use a written log to track medication. Others may use a computer-based student medical record system. Either system works well as long as it is kept consistently. A monthly log is provided in Appendix 8.

On the log, note how many pills (or how much liquid) the school was given. When the pill bottle is finished, the number of recorded administrations should be equal to the number of pills. If a discrepancy exists, steps must be taken to account for the missing medication. The log system will also allow the school to notify families when medications need to be refilled. Keep in mind that some medications prescribed for children are controlled substances. This means that prescriptions cannot be called in to the pharmacy. Families need notice well before medications run out.

Errors in medication administration or in log keeping are almost inevitable. We recommend that one person be designated to monitor errors (usually the school nurse). If an error is made, that person should be notified immediately. Part of this person's job should be to monitor patterns of errors and take steps to prevent future errors from occurring. For example, if a child consistently misses a dose of medication from being out of class for therapy, a new system needs to be put in place to ensure that the child receives medication on therapy days as well. For this type of system to work, it is essential that errors be dealt with in a manner that encourages reporting of errors. In most circumstances, staff should be rewarded, not punished, for reporting errors. Punishment should be reserved for times when school employees act with malice or gross negligence or consistently make errors.

LEGAL ISSUES

Parents and school officials often express confusion over what the law dictates about medications and schools. Nine of the most common questions about medications and the law are answered below.

1. *Are there any federal or state laws about medication in schools?* Section 504 of the Rehabilitation Act of 1973 and Title II of the Americans with Disabilities Act state that children should not be discriminated against on the basis of disability. These laws require schools to make reasonable accommodations for students with disabilities, and reasonable accommodations for some students may include the provision of medications. Some states have also passed laws or guidelines that are more specific than this act and should be consulted as well. School boards and superintendents are usually required to follow the policies set in place by federal and state law. When situations arise that are not addressed in federal or state guidelines, then it is the responsibility of the school board to seek legal and medical advice to establish a policy.

2. *Given all the liabilities associated with medications, can the school refuse to administer medication?* Public schools cannot refuse to administer medications prescribed for chronic health conditions (including disabilities such as ADHD and depression). Section 504 states that schools must provide accommodations for the needs of children with health conditions. This means that the school must provide assistance to meet the needs of the child and therefore cannot refuse to administer medication.

3. *Can we require the child's parent to administer medications?* Schools receiving federal funding are mandated to provide needed medications to children with chronic health conditions. This means that they cannot require that parents come to school to administer medication. Similarly, the school cannot refuse to provide medication due to limited resources. These laws do not usually bind private schools that do not receive federal funding.

4. *Can we refuse to administer herbal remedies?* Herbal and over-the-counter medications can be problematic for schools. Some of these medications are associated with unknown or serious side effects. The safest thing to do is to treat herbal and over-the-counter medications like prescription medications, which is to require a note from the child's physician that indicates that the child needs be given these medications. The physician should be asked to provide the same information about these medications as prescription information: name, dose, when to administer, possible side effects, and so on.

5. *Does the law require that a registered nurse provide medication to children?* No, although a school nurse is the ideal person to administer medication at school. This is not always practical or possible in today's economy. It was once common for each school to have a full-time nurse, but many schools today have a nurse only part time or don't have a nurse at all. If a school nurse is not available to supervise the provision of medication, an alternative staff member can be designated. The person who is designated to give medication should be trained to administer the medication properly and taught how to handle problems. Even when school nurses are available to provide medication, there may be times when an alternate adult needs to be designated to provide medication. For example, the parents and school can work together to determine how best to provide medication on days when the child is not on school grounds, such as field-trip days.

6. *Should medication administration be a part of the child's 504 plan?* Yes, in most cases, medication administration will be part of the child's 504 plan.

7. *Are privacy issues addressed in the law?* Yes, the HIPAA (Health Insurance Portability and Accountability Act, 1996) and the FERPA (Family Educational Rights and Pri-

vacy Act, 1974; see also National Association of School Nurses, 2000; National Task Force on Confidential Student Health Information, 2000) ensure a student's right to confidentiality. A child's medical information must be carefully protected because the child and family deserve this privacy and because the school, district, and state may face serious lawsuits if confidentiality is violated.

8. *Can older students carry their own medication to school?* In some cases, yes. In a few cases, some schools or districts can make decisions whether to grant students permission to transport medications. For adolescents who use medications that are not controlled substances, this may be a desirable arrangement. If the medications are controlled substances, the student must be deemed sufficiently responsible to remember to carry a daily dose to school and take it as prescribed. This decision should be made jointly between parents and school staff.

9. *Whose responsibility is it to make sure a child's medications have been taken?* It is the school's responsibility to make sure that a child takes medications provided to the school. If a child consistently forgets to take medication, then a new system needs to be devised to prevent such errors.

ATTITUDES TOWARD MEDICATIONS

Many families are reluctant to use medications and may prefer behavior therapy to medication management. Families can first explore ways to manage the child's behavior through environmental changes and manipulations. In fact, for many professionals, tried-and-true techniques such as positive reinforcement, time-out, and response cost are the preferred first line of treatment.

Some families may not be ready to commit to an intervention of any kind. If you believe you are dealing with this type of family, it can be helpful to ask parents if they believe that their child has a problem and have them describe exactly what they think the problem is. Families who report that their child does not have any problems or only very minor problems are unlikely to seek treatment. If they are persuaded to seek treatment in spite of their belief that no problem exists, they may be unlikely to follow through on the physician's recommendations. For families who deny that their child has any type of problem, it can be helpful to start by documenting observations about the child and sharing these observations with the family. Letting them know you think their child is suffering and you want to make the child's world better is also helpful. Providing the family with resources so they can learn about childhood disorders and treatments may result in good, informed decisions about treatment for the child. These families need a great deal of emotional support during this process.

Nancy is a 6-year-old first grader. Her teacher has been concerned about symptoms of inattention and impulsivity that are significantly affecting her academic performance. Nancy is having a hard time making friends because she is impulsive and often is too rough or is insensitive toward other children. When Nancy's teacher, Ms. Dennison, brought these concerns up to Nancy's parents, they at first adamantly denied that Nancy's behavior was a problem at home. Over the next 2 weeks, Ms. Dennison kept careful records of Nancy's behavior and collected several work samples. She recorded the amount of time it took Nancy to complete worksheets and compared it to the rest of the class. Because she knew that Nancy's family was active in their church and trusted their minister, she also suggested that they talk to their minister and to Nancy's Sunday school teacher to see if similar problems had been observed in other environments. When Nancy's parents returned 2 weeks later for a follow-up confer- ence, they reported that other adults in Nancy's life also felt she had a problem. How- ever, they were reluctant to bring her to the physician because they "don't believe in medication for children." Ms. Dennison counseled them, "Why don't you make an appointment with your physician to have Nancy evaluated. There are lots of different things that can cause a child to have a hard time at school. Once you know why Nancy is having a hard time, your physician will be able to talk to you about the choices you have to help her. Often, the first choices are not medication choices. By consulting your physician, you'll know what the best treatment is, depending on the diagnosis. You won't know what options you have until you talk to the physician, and I know you want what's best for her in the long run."

Even families that have accepted that their child has a problem and have sought help may require support to ensure treatment adherence. Factors such as side effects, costs, social acceptability, and beliefs that the medication is helping can exert significant control over the likelihood that a child will continue to take medication as prescribed by the physi- cian. It is important to remind families that they should talk to the physician if they have concerns about their child's treatment before deciding to abandon treatment altogether. The provider may be able to prescribe a medication that is less costly, has a less demanding administration schedule, or has fewer side effects. If a medication is having positive effects on the child's academic, behavioral, or social life, it is important that these observations be shared with the child's family.

Despite the documented efficacy of many psychotropic medications for children, the use of these medications continues to be controversial. Opponents argue that medications do not solve the underlying cause of problems, or they believe that medications are used inappropriately to solve problems that could be treated through nonmedical interventions. Both concerns are valid. Psychotropic medications for children do not cure the cause of behavioral and emotional problems in children. Instead, they treat the symptoms of these problems. Additionally, there almost certainly are cases where children are inappropriately prescribed medication before other less intrusive forms of intervention are attempted. When parents have these concerns, the best response is often to encourage them to talk to their physician or others about their concerns or to seek a second opinion.

If parents refuse to seek treatment for their child and the child's problems are very severe, it may be necessary is to lodge a charge of medical neglect with the department of social services (or equivalent state agency) in your state. Medical neglect means that mini- mal health care is not being obtained for the child and that the negligence may lead to seri- ous harm or death. For example, if you believe a child has an eating disorder, but the family refuses to seek any type of treatment, it is possible the child may eventually die from the condition, and a medical-neglect charge should be made while the child is still healthy. Similar arguments can be made when children are very depressed or self-injurious.

Remember that as a professional who cares for children, you are mandated to make a report if you believe that child abuse or neglect is taking place. This may be difficult but is essential for the welfare of the child. If you suspect that the child is being medically neglected but you are not sure, it is appropriate and sometimes mandated to call the department of social services and make the report. This gives the agency the chance to decide whether or not to accept the report and takes the decision-making responsibility away from the school personnel. Unfortunately, policies and standards vary from state to state and from county to county within a state. If you are unclear about policies or laws in your state, advocate for your school system to hold training sessions that will clarify them. Again, the welfare of the child is the goal of all school providers and other professionals.

TREATMENT ACCEPTABILITY

Some children are resistant to taking medications. Some may have social concerns about letting others know of their problem. Others may object to the way the medication tastes or the side effects of the medication. The following strategies can increase treatment acceptability among children.

For the Child Who Is Embarrassed to Take Medications

The first step in solving this problem is to ask the child what he or she wants to do. Then talk to the child and parents about what is okay for other children to know about the medication and the child's situation. Some children may be comfortable about other children knowing that they take a medication to help them pay attention better but may be less comfortable about others knowing that a medication is used for tics. If the child continues to be embarrassed about taking medication, have the child decide on a secret signal (e.g., a hand signal or a teacher's watch that beeps) that alerts teacher and child that it is medication time. Let the child know that if the response to the signal is quick enough, the teacher will not have to remind him or her about the medication:

"Mary, when I give you a thumbs-up sign, that means that you are excused to go take your medication. As long as you get up and go right away, I won't need to remind you about it. That way, you can keep this information to yourself more easily."

Another option is to consider allowing the child to do a special job for the class each day when it is time to take medications. For example, a child who needs to take a medication at 11:00 A.M. each day can be given the job of taking the attendance sheet down to the office at 10:55. Medication can be taken at the office after delivering the attendance sheet.

For the Child Who Is Resistant to Taking Medications

Children who resist taking medications are not necessarily oppositional or trying to cause problems. Be aware that some children resist taking medications because the taste is terrible or they have uncomfortable side effects. In addition, taking time out to take medication can sometimes mean missing out on part of a fun activity. Start by making a behavioral contract with the child that is signed by the child, teacher, and parents (Appendix 9). Each day, allow the child to earn a specified number of points for taking the medication. Points can be tracked with pennies in a jar, a sticker sheet, or a "checkbook." Once the child earns the agreed number of points, the points can be taken home and redeemed for a reward. If you are concerned the child's family may not be able to follow through on this type of reward system, classroom privileges such as a homework pass can also be used. Figure 2.3 is an example of a medication contract that was used for Donna Wang, a 6-year-old girl who was prescribed medication to manage a tic disorder that she had recently developed. During the first week of medication, Donna's school nurse noticed that she was spending a lot of time trying to get Donna to take her medication because it "tasted yucky." She decided to try a behavioral contract in which Donna could earn up to a half hour per week of library time for taking her medication without complaining. Because Donna loved library time, the intervention worked well starting on the first day. In fact, Donna and the school nurse were able to make a game out of not complaining in which they joked about how wonderful the medication tasted and how she couldn't wait to take it. Donna's mother was so impressed that she designed a similar reward system at home to help Donna take her medication without complaining.

I, _Donna Wang_ , agree to take my medication every day
at _11:30_ A.M./P.M.

I will earn 1 point each time I take my medication.

When I earn _5_ points, I will receive
A 30-minute library pass to use when Ms. Laural says it is OK.

Child's signature: _Donna Wang_
Parent's signature: _Carol Wang_
School personnel signature: _Ms. Laural_

FIGURE 2.3. Example of completed medication contract.

For the Child Who Pretends to Take Medications

With any medication taken at school, it is important to keep a pill count (see Appendix 8 for a sample pill log). You may need to supervise the child carefully. You can also ask parents to talk to the child's physician about alternative methods of administration. Some children are resistant to taking liquid medication because it tastes bad but are willing to take it in pill form. On the other hand, a child who frequently gags while taking pills may start to resist medication. A liquid form may be more appropriate in this case.

For the Child Who Gets Sick When Trying to Swallow a Pill

The physician can work with the child on ways to make pill swallowing easier. Giving rewards for successful swallowing is useful. Some capsules can be opened and sprinkled into pudding or applesauce. The child's physician must approve this procedure because it can be dangerous to break up some types of pills. Some children need to be taught the mechanics of pill swallowing. They can be shown a picture of the digestive system and the flap that closes over the windpipe when they swallow. This flap covers the windpipe so that the pill can only go down the esophagus. Pill swallowing can be made easier by simple strategies like taking a few drinks before trying to take the pill to lubricate the throat and placing the pill far back in the mouth before trying to swallow it. In rare cases, children have a serious phobia about pill swallowing and will require desensitization training with a health professional. Parents need to be aware that there are treatments available to make pill swallowing easier so that each administration is not a battle.

For the Child Who Is Very Thirsty Because of the Medication

Some teachers may choose to give the child with excessive thirst a continual free pass to the drinking fountain. An alternative to assigning drinking fountain privileges to just one child is to consider allowing all children in your class to keep a water bottle in their desk or backpack so they can drink when they need to without disrupting the rest of the class. This method would also offer the child the option to take medication discreetly.

For the Child Who Needs to Use the Restroom Frequently and Immediately Due to Medication Side Effects

Make an agreement with the child to use the restroom at specified times during the day with as much volume as possible, even if the child does not think it seems necessary at the time. The child can agree to try to use the restroom before coming to class, at the end of the morning recess, at the end of lunch, and at the beginning of silent reading time. Scheduling bathroom breaks at appropriate times (e.g., transitions, at the end of recess) will help prevent the child from making emergency trips during instructional times. It also helps the child maintain dignity. It may be necessary to have the child sign a reward contract similar to the medication contract to encourage specific and frequent restroom breaks.

For the Child Who Refuses to Eat

Some medications exert an effect on appetite and significantly decrease a child's appetite while receiving medication. Let the child's parents know if the child is not eating lunch. The child may be eating enough at other times of the day to compensate, but in these cases it is important that the child's family monitor food intake and that the child's physician monitor weight gain and health status. It may be helpful to send the child's uneaten lunch home so parents have an idea of what is being eaten. Also, work with parents to find a food that the child is willing to eat at lunchtime. For example, some children will eat yogurt and a granola bar even when they can't eat a sandwich. If the child is not eating and is becoming disruptive during the lunch hour, assign a constructive activity while the other children eat. Some children enjoy being given jobs to do during lunchtime (e.g., helping cafeteria workers serve food). Others might enjoy having crayons or a book.

SUMMARY

Despite the difficulties and liabilities associated with medications, medications allow freedom. Children who might have previously required hospitalization may now be treated and managed while attending school. Children who might have previously failed classes may now graduate from high school and even go on to college. Children who might have previously hated school or had few friends may now have positive educational or social experiences. School personnel are important partners in the medical management of children with emotional, behavioral, and learning problems. School personnel are often the first to recognize that a problem exists and can provide information and support for families who are seeking treatment. They can provide important information about how the child performs in a structured environment, how the child compares to others of the same age, and how the child behaves socially. They can also monitor learning and behavior to help physicians make decisions about treatment choices. These contributions make a treatment plan far more likely to be successful.

REFERENCES

Family Educational Rights and Privacy Act. (1974). 20 U.S.C. §1231g; 34 CFR, Part 99.

Health Insurance Portability and Accountability Act. (1996). Public Law No. 104-191.

National Association of School Nurses. (2000). *Guidelines for protecting confidential student health information*. Scarborough, ME: Author.

National Task Force on Confidential Student Health Information. (2000). *Guidelines for protecting confidential student health information*. Kent, OH: American School Health Association.

3

Classifications of Psychotropic Medications

It is helpful to discuss medications in terms of the classes they fall into because medications in the same class tend to have similar treatment effects, side effects, risk factors, and interactions. Categories of side effects are associated with certain medication classes. Several types of side effects that may be associated with psychiatric medications are described in Table 3.1. Comparison of medications within a class is also helpful because individual medications may have advantages or disadvantages when compared to other medications in the same class.

TABLE 3.1. Description of Side Effects

Side effect	Description
Anticholinergic	Dry mouth, cognitive impairment, blurred vision, constipation
Agranulocytosis	Toxicity of the bone marrow resulting in white blood count depletion; requires weekly blood monitoring
Akathisia	Feelings of restlessness, muscle tension, foot tapping, and rocking from side to side; may include apathy and lack of facial expression
Acute dystonia	Severe motor spasms of the jaw, neck, tongue, and back
Akinesia	Impaired body movement
Extrapyramidal symptoms	Acute dystonia, akathisia, akinesia, and Parkinsonian side effects
Neuroleptic malignant syndrome	A potentially fatal syndrome including exceptionally high fever, rigidity, unstable pulse and blood pressures, and altered consciousness
Parkinsonian side effects	Arm swing, slow motor movement, rigidity, slow speech, lack of movement in facial expression
Serotonin syndrome	Potentially life-threatening reaction characterized by mental confusion, agitation, shivering, tremor, diarrhea, incoordination, and fever
Tardive dyskinesia	Abnormal involuntary movement of the mouth, face, tongue, and neck; may be irreversible

We chose to discuss classification of psychotropic medications because medications in the same class are often used to treat similar disorders. Table 3.2 reviews the types of medicines used with schoolchildren. Medications in the same class are believed to affect the brain in similar ways, but medications in different classes work in different ways. For example, selective serotonin reuptake inhibitors (SSRIs) and tricyclics are both prescribed to treat depression, but they work in different ways by affecting different chemicals (neurotransmitters) in the brain. Although medications in the same class are often used to treat similar disorders, the same class of medications may be used to treat many types of problems. Medications known as antipsychotics, for example, are not used just for psychotic symptoms like hallucinations and delusions. They may also be effective in treating some types of mood disorders, tic disorders, and severe aggression.

In this chapter, we discuss stimulant, antidepressant, anxiolytic (antianxiety), mood stabilizer, neuroleptic (antipsychotic), and antihypertensive classes of medication. For each class of medication, we provide a brief overview of the class brand and generic names. The treatment effects, possible side effects, potential interactions with other substances and medications, and any potential for abuse or misuse are also detailed.

STIMULANTS

Stimulant medications are the most commonly prescribed psychotropic medications for children. This is because of the number of children diagnosed with ADHD and the effectiveness of this class of medications with ADHD symptoms. More research has been conducted on stimulant medications than on any other medication class for children. Stimulants work by making it easier for certain neurons to talk to other neurons in the child's brain. All of the stimulants have similar effects, but different stimulant medications can work in a variety of ways and to different degrees to reduce ADHD symptoms. The most common stimulants prescribed to children include methylphenidate, dextroamphetamine, and amphetamine compounds like Adderall.

It is clear that stimulant medications are effective for the treatment of such ADHD symptoms as hyperactivity, inattention, and impulsivity. Studies showing the beneficial effects of stimulant medications have been conducted in a number of ways: laboratory tests, natural observation at home and at school, and checklists completed by parents and

TABLE 3.2. Classifications of Psychotropic Medications for Children

Class	Common problems
Stimulant	Hyperactivity, inattention, impulsivity
Antidepressant	Depression, anxiety, obsessive–compulsive disorder, tic disorders, bedwetting
Anxiolytic	Anxiety, panic disorder
Mood stabilizer	Bipolar disorder, severe mood swings, seizures
Neuroleptic	Hallucinations, delusions, tic disorders, self-injury, aggression
Antihypertensive	Tic disorders, ADHD, aggression, self-injury

teachers. Stimulant medications can result in improvements in attention, school performance, and social success. Stimulant use is also associated with improved interactions with parents, peers, and teachers. Research findings are summarized in Table 3.3.

Despite excellent research support for the use of stimulants for treatment of hyperactivity, inattention, and impulsivity, their use continues to be controversial. Historically, parents and medical personnel thought these medications might make a child more likely to commit crimes or to abuse illegal substances later in life. We now know the use of stimulant medication may in fact help children avoid such negative life pathways. Another concern a few years ago was that the long-term use of stimulants caused growth problems. This concern has not been substantiated by research. A few children taking stimulants do experience a considerable decrease in appetite. Failure to eat is likely to cause weight loss that in turn may impair growth. For this small group of children, physicians will monitor the effects of medication and may change the dose or change to a new medication.

Sustained-Release Stimulants

Stimulants are short-acting drugs. This means their effect usually peaks between 1 and 4 hours after consumption. This short half-life means that multiple doses may need to be taken throughout the day. Parents are sometimes concerned about potential problems with their child taking doses at school. The child may not remember the dose. If the child feels stigmatized leaving the classroom to go to the school nurse for medication, the school dose may be avoided. The child's peers may perceive the child as different and perhaps tease and embarrass the child. Teachers may also be concerned about disruption in the flow of work for children and classmates. For these reasons, the sustained-release stimulants are becoming more popular. Sustained-release stimulants simply extend the release of the shorter-acting stimulants. Four types are Ritalin LA (long acting), Concerta, Metadate, and

TABLE 3.3. Beneficial Effects of Stimulant Medications

Type of effect	Research findings
Cognitive	Better performance on tasks requiring vigilance and sustained attention More efficient cognitive strategies to find items Improvement on stimulus-reaction timed tasks Enhanced performance on recall tasks Improved paired-associate learning Improved performance on tasks requiring perceptual and motor function Enhanced receptive language capacity and auditory processing skills
Academic	Improved performance on schoolwork Improved classroom behavior More work attempted Increased percentage of correct answers More on-task performance
Behavioral	Improvements in rule-governed behavior Improved compliance with adult commands Decreased physical and verbal aggression Improved interactions with parents, siblings, teachers, and peers

Adderall XR (extended release). These medications usually need to be taken only once per day, and the child can take the medication at home before coming to school. Some parents are more comfortable with this arrangement because privacy is maintained and they have control over their child's medications. Nonetheless, parents should be encouraged to let the school know what medications their child is taking, even when those medications are not administered at school.

The absorption rates of longer-acting medications are less predictable, and the child may experience some unevenness in the drug's effectiveness during the school day and in after-school activities. Some parents also find that their child's long-acting stimulant wears off during the critical homework hour. When this happens, the child's physician may decide to alternate or mix different stimulants or their release versions. To help physicians achieve the right balance for each child, feedback from educators, coaches, and other school personnel needs to be added to feedback from parents. For the greatest benefit in designing medication regimens and behavioral programs, the child's behavior and attention should be described in a variety of situations and over time.

Some people believe a child can be diagnosed as having ADHD if the child behaves better when taking a stimulant. Unfortunately, this approach is not effective. Although many children with ADHD respond to stimulants, about one fourth to one third do not respond as successfully to these medications. Additionally, sometimes children who do not have ADHD are more attentive and have an easier time focusing when they take stimulants. This type of response is sometimes normal and does not necessarily mean that the child has a disability or needs medication.

Side Effects

Table 3.4 outlines side effects of several stimulants. The most usual short-term side effects of stimulants are insomnia and appetite suppression. Some children who are taking stimulant medications may not be hungry at lunchtime. When this happens, it is important to assess the child's food intake and alert the parents. The child may be compensating for the lack of lunch appetite with bigger breakfasts or dinners. However, parents need to know that lunch is being skipped so they can encourage the child to eat

TABLE 3.4. Common Side Effects of Stimulant Medications

Generic name	Trade name	Common side effects
Amphetamine	Adderall	Decreased appetite, insomnia, abdominal pain, emotional ups and downs
Dextroamphetamine	Dexedrine	Restlessness, constipation or diarrhea, dizziness, dry mouth, headache, heart palpitations, high blood pressure, decreased appetite, sleeplessness, stomach and intestinal disturbances, tremors, unpleasant taste in the mouth, weight loss
Methylphenidate	Concerta, Metadate, Ritalin	Sleep problems, nervousness, decreased appetite, abdominal pain, weight loss, sleep problems, fast heartbeat

more at other times of the day, and teachers can encourage the child to eat more at lunch or snack time.

Stimulant side effects that occur less frequently are irritability, sadness, moodiness, agitation, and dizziness. Tearfulness can be a sign that the medication is not a good choice for a child.

Some children experience an increase in ADHD symptoms beyond baseline when the medication wears off. This is known as a rebound effect and may indicate a need for a change or adjustment in the child's medication regimen. The child's physician should address the problem. Lack of any effect or negative side effects usually indicate a need for a medication change.

Not responding well to one stimulant does not mean that a child will not respond well to a different stimulant or that a different type of medication would not be of benefit. Many children with ADHD are prescribed several medications before one that is effective for them is identified. For this reason, the child's physician may ask school personnel to provide multiple reports about the child's behavior over the course of the school year. These reports are used to make decisions about whether a medication is working and whether medication changes are needed.

Some children who take stimulant medications develop tics. Tics are repetitive motor movements (such as eye blinking) or sounds (such as throat clearing). It is not clear whether the medications actually cause tics or whether they make tics more noticeable in children who were already prone to them. If tics are noticeable only when the child is taking a stimulant medication, the physician may choose a different class of medication to treat the child's ADHD, perhaps antihypertensives or antidepressants.

Dosage and Interaction with Other Drugs

It is not usually dangerous for a child to miss a dose of a stimulant medication. A missed dose will typically result only in more noticeable symptoms of ADHD. However, the medication should be given as close to the prescribed time as possible to ensure maximum benefit. This is especially true when a child is taking multiple types of medications at multiple times during the day. If a child is more than 1 hour late taking a stimulant medication, the parent should be contacted so a decision can be made whether to take the dose late or skip the dose altogether. Some children have a difficult time sleeping at night if they take their medication late in the day. In some cases, then, it may be preferable to skip the dose rather than take it late in the day. Talk to parents in advance about their preferences.

When tricyclic antidepressants (discussed later in this chapter) and decongestants like Sudafed are taken with stimulants, the effects of both the stimulant and the second medication can be enhanced. Be aware that this enhancement of effects can result in unwanted side effects. On the other hand, antihistamines like Benadryl can decrease the effectiveness of the stimulants, causing the medication to appear as if it is not working. Teachers and parents should know that Cylert has been associated with liver problems and requires blood tests to monitor liver functioning. The other stimulants do not normally require regular blood tests.

Precautions

The federal Drug Enforcement Administration (DEA) considers most stimulants to be substances that have a high risk for abuse. They are categorized as schedule II drugs. This means that the prescription must be handwritten and hand-signed by the physician and the medication is highly regulated by the DEA. The parent must get the written prescription at the physician's office because schedule II medication prescriptions cannot be phoned in to a pharmacy.

When taken as prescribed by the person for whom they were prescribed, stimulants pose little risk for abuse. A serious cautionary note, however, is that stimulants may be used inappropriately or may be used by an individual other than the one for whom the prescription was intended. Sometimes other members of the child's family may take the child's stimulants to help them stay awake and alert. In other cases, the medication may be taken in a method different from that prescribed (e.g., crushed and snorted) by either the child or by a friend or family member. Some teenagers discover they can sell their medications to friends. If these medications are being stored at school, they must be carefully monitored. Some physicians are reluctant to prescribe additional medication for a child when a pill bottle has been lost or stolen. In a very high percentage of cases, these medications are used as they were intended and by the individual for whom they were intended. At the same time, school personnel can help ferret out unscrupulous stimulant medication activities.

ANTIDEPRESSANTS

Antidepressant medications are traditionally used to treat depression in adults. They also have been used to treat a variety of childhood disorders, including mood disorders, anxiety disorders, obsessive–compulsive disorder, ADHD, tic disorders, and bedwetting. There are four major classes of antidepressants: SSRIs, tricyclics, monoamine oxidase inhibitors (MAOIs), and atypical antidepressants. Table 3.5 provides a brief overview of each of these classes of medications. Each class of antidepressant has different ways of affecting the brain, resulting in different clinical effects. Table 3.6 is a summary of common side effects seen in several antidepressants that are used with children.

TABLE 3.5. Classes of Antidepressant Medications

Type	How they work	Advantages and disadvantages
SSRI	Decreases reabsorption (reuptake) of serotonin so serotonin levels in the brain are increased.	Fewer side effects than other antidepressants, can cause mania or agitation.
Tricyclic	Affects levels of various neurotransmitters in the brain.	Overdose can be lethal, side effects such as dry mouth and sedation can be significant.
MAOI	Prevents norepinephrine and dopamine from being broken down.	Significant dietary restrictions that must be followed.
Atypical	Affects levels of several neurotransmitters.	Varies.

TABLE 3.6. Common Side Effects of Antidepressant Medications

Generic name	Trade name	Common side effects
SSRIs		
Fluoxetine	Prozac	Anxiety, nervousness
Sertraline	Zoloft	Diarrhea, dizziness, drowsiness, dry mouth, headache, indigestion, fatigue, insomnia, nausea, nervousness, tingling, or vomiting
Fluvoxamine	Luvox	Decreased appetite, constipation, dry mouth, headache, nausea, nervousness, skin rash, sleep problems, sleepiness
Paroxetine	Paxil	Constipation or diarrhea, decreased appetite, dizziness, drowsiness, dry mouth, nausea, nervousness, sleeplessness, sweating, tremor, weakness, vertigo
Citalopram	Celexa	Abdominal pain, agitation, anxiety, diarrhea, drowsiness, dry mouth, fatigue, indigestion, insomnia, loss of appetite, nausea, sweating, tremor, vomiting
Tricyclics		
Desipramine	Norpramin, Pertofrane	Dry mouth, visual disturbance, constipation, dizziness, drowsiness, increased perspiration, mild tremors, insomnia
Nortriptyline	Pamelor, Vivactil	Headache, nausea, sweating, dry mouth, sleepiness or insomnia, diarrhea or constipation, blurry vision, weight gain
Imipramine	Tofranil	Nervousness, sleep disorders, stomach problems, tiredness, anxiety, constipation, convulsions, emotional ups and downs, fainting
Amitriptyline	Elavil	Vision problems, constipation, difficulty urinating, dry mouth, fatigue, sensitivity to sunlight, temperature sensitivity
Clomipramine	Anafranil	Vision problems, constipation, drowsiness, dry mouth, low blood pressure, nausea, vomiting
Atypical		
Venlafaxine	Effexor	Anxiety, constipation, depression, difficulty breathing, dizziness, dry mouth, itching, loss of appetite, weakness, nausea, nervousness, sedation, skin rash, sleep problems, sweating, tingling hands or feet, tremors, vomiting, strange dreams, weight loss
Trazodone	Desyrel	Dizziness, drowsiness, lightheadedness
Bupropion	Wellbutrin	Abdominal pain, agitation, anxiety, constipation, dizziness, dry mouth, excessive sweating, headache, loss of appetite, nausea, palpitations, vomiting, skin rash, sleep disturbances, sore throat, tremor
Mirtazapine	Remeron	Strange dreams and thoughts, constipation, dizziness, dry mouth, flu-like symptoms, increased appetite, sleepiness, weakness, weight gain

Selective Serotonin Reuptake Inhibitors

SSRIs are the most widely prescribed type of antidepressant medication for children. They include fluoxetine, sertraline, citalopram, paroxetine, and fluvoxamine. SSRIs work on the neurons that release the neurotransmitter called serotonin. SSRIs prevent these releaser cells from reabsorbing (reuptaking) the serotonin once it has been released. As a result, more serotonin is available for a longer time to the brain cells that need it.

SSRIs can be effective in treating symptoms of obsessive–compulsive disorder, ADHD, and selective mutism in children. They are often used to treat other anxiety and mood disorders in children, although their effectiveness in treating these disorders in children has not been explored thoroughly. The full effect of an SSRI may not occur for 4 to 8 weeks.

SSRIs are associated with fewer side effects than other types of antidepressants but there are some. These include irritability, agitation, headaches, insomnia, diarrhea, stomachaches, and sedation. SSRIs affect the ability of the liver to process other medications, including common over-the-counter products, so parents need to consult the child's physician before giving other medications.

In some cases, the use of SSRIs can induce manic or hypomanic episodes. Symptoms can include extreme loss of control of behavior, agitation, feelings of euphoria, and excitability. This problem is relatively rare and may occur when children are prescribed high doses or when they are at risk for bipolar disorder. There has also been concern that some SSRIs may cause violent or suicidal thoughts and behaviors in some children. The first signs of risk behavior typically occur during the first three weeks of medication treatment. Early signs include onset of significant agitation and irritability. Right now, it is not clear whether a real association between SSRIs and these symptoms exists. However, the FDA has recently required drug manufacturers to place "black box" warning labels on all SSRIs. The labels warn that in some children, these medications have been linked to depression and suicide. Appendix 10 includes the wording recommended by the FDA for its black box warnings, as well as a list of antidepressants now on the market that carry these warning labels.Prozac is the only SSRI approved for use by children. The child's physician should be knowledgeable about the most recent studies and will decide if the benefits of the medication are greater than possible risks. The best advice is that anytime a child has a disorder such as depression or anxiety, it is prudent to supervise the child and closely monitor changes in mood and behavior, regardless of the type of treatment prescribed.

Some SSRIs are available in short-acting and long-acting forms. Physicians often prefer short-acting forms because they are easier to discontinue if unacceptable side effects arise. However, the long-acting forms can be helpful when a child has difficulty remembering to take medication.

If a child misses a dose of an SSRI, the dose should be taken as soon as it is remembered and the parent should be contacted. Two doses should not be given at the same time. If several doses are missed, the child may suffer from such symptoms as dizziness, nausea, fatigue, sleep disturbance, anxiety, moodiness, and irritability. When SSRIs are discontinued by a physician, they are done so gradually. Children should not stop taking SSRIs abruptly. Discontinuation should be initiated only after consulting the child's physician.

Tricyclic Antidepressants

Tricylic antidepressants (TCAs) affect multiple neurotransmitters in the brain, including serotonin, dopamine, and norepinephrine. TCAs include amitriptyline, imipramine, desipramine, nortriptyline, doxepin, clomipramine, and protriptyline.

TCAs are frequently used to treat depression in adults, but in children, they are used to treat disorders such as bedwetting, ADHD, and Tourette's disorder. Because they are somewhat sedating, TCAs can decrease impulsiveness, hyperactivity, inattention, and anxiety. They also can help to improve cooperation from some children. In addition, because they usually are not associated with tics, they can be helpful when a child with ADHD experiences unacceptable or intolerable increases in tics from stimulants. Low doses of

TCAs are also used to treat bedwetting. However, the treatment usually works only while the child is taking the medication, and bedwetting often recurs when the child stops taking the medication. TCAs may also be used to alleviate depression and anxiety disorders in children and adolescents, although research is still needed to determine how well these medications work for these age groups.

The negative side effects associated with TCAs, and especially the risk of overdose, make them a second or third treatment choice for many childhood disorders. Sedation is the most common side effect seen with the TCAs. Other side effects are drowsiness, dizziness, lethargy, dry mouth, tremors, sleep problems, nausea, constipation, stomachaches, chest pains, palpitations, blurred vision, and perspiration. These side effects can cause difficulty in the classroom. Children who are taking TCAs may need to take frequent water fountain breaks or bring bottled water to class to counteract mouth dryness. They may also need frequent access to a restroom because of their increased fluid intake. Some children may get a red and itchy rash that usually appears on the chest. This rash is not usually serious, but parents should be alerted when it occurs so that they can tell the child's physician.

The greatest risk with TCAs is overdose. Children taking TCAs can die from accidental or intended overdose. If a child who is taking a TCA shows a change in mental status (does not seem to be thinking right or is behaving strangely), passes out, or has a seizure, an ambulance should be called and medical personnel should be alerted that the child is taking a TCA and may be experiencing an overdose. Because the risk for overdose is so great, physicians often elect to prescribe TCAs only when parents can provide assurance that the medication will be strictly monitored.

If a child is late taking a TCA dose at school, the dose should be taken as soon as it is remembered and the parents should be told the time the medication was taken. However, if a dose has been missed entirely (not remembered), never give two doses at the same time. This can result in a fatal overdose. If the child misses multiple doses, symptoms such as headache and stomach problems may occur.

Monoamine Oxidase Inhibitors

MAOIs are among the oldest and most effective antidepressants. However, because of the dietary restrictions associated with these medications, they are rarely used in children. Therefore, we present only a very brief overview of these medications. MAOIs include phenelzine, isocarboxazid, and tranylcypromine. MAOIs work by preventing chemicals called monoamines from being released in the brain. This in turn increases the availability of multiple neurotransmitters in the brain. A major concern for children on these drugs is adverse interaction with other elements. These include foods containing the amino acid tyramine (found in most cheeses), drugs of abuse, and most cold medications. When consumed with an MAOI, each of these substances can raise blood pressure to a dangerously high level. Some short-term negative effects of MAOIs include weight gain, drowsiness, dizziness, and swings in blood pressure. The diet of any child taking an MAOI will need to be monitored with vigilance. Most children will be instructed to eat only food that has been sent from home and to avoid food prepared in the school cafeteria.

Atypical Antidepressants

The atypical antidepressants include bupropion, trazodone, mirtazapine, and venlafaxine. We refer to these substances as atypical antidepressants because they affect the brain a little bit differently from other antidepressants. For example, bupropion affects the neurotransmitter called dopamine, and venlafaxine affects the neurotransmitters called serotonin and norepinephrine.

Bupropion has been used to treat ADHD, aggression, and depression. It is also used to help teenagers and adults quit smoking (marketed as Zyban). Bupropion can cause insomnia, loss of appetite, irritability, and sometimes an increase in tics. This medication may also make a child susceptible to seizures. Bupropion should not be used with adolescents who have bulimia because it may put them at greater risk of having a seizure. Venlafaxine is sometimes used to treat children with depression and obsessive–compulsive disorder. Side effects can include nausea, headaches, and blood pressure elevation. Trazadone are used for sleep problems, anxiety, depression, and oppositional behaviors. At high doses, these medications may cause agitation, sedation, constipation, dry mouth, and confusion. Mirtazapine is often used for children who have difficulty falling asleep and who have symptoms of depression. Side effects can include fatigue and gastrointestinal difficulties.

You should consult a child's parents ahead of time as to what they want the school to do if the child is late taking a dose of an atypical antidepressant. In some cases, the child should be given the medication as soon as it is remembered. In other cases, the dose will need to be skipped. A child should not be given two doses at the same time.

ANXIOLYTICS

Anxiolytics are used to treat anxiety disorders, described as conditions that are generally manifested by symptoms of nervousness, worrying, or panic. This class of medicines includes benzodiazepines, antihistamines, and buspirone. An overview of selected anxiolytics and their side effects is presented in Table 3.7.

TABLE 3.7. Common Side Effects of Anxiolytic Medications

Generic name	Trade name	Common side effects
Clonazepam	Klonopin	Anxiety, behavior problems, insomnia, irritability, drowsiness, problems with coordination
Alprazolam	Xanax	Clumsiness, sleepiness
Triazolam	Halcion	Clumsiness, sleepiness
Lorazepam	Ativan	Clumsiness, dizziness, sleepiness, unsteadiness, weakness
Diazepam	Valium	Clumsiness, sleepiness
Clorazepate	Tranxene	Clumsiness, sleepiness
Chlordiazepoxide	Librium	Clumsiness, sleepiness

Benzodiazepines

Benzodiazepines are considered to be sedative medications. This means that they may make the child more calm or sleepy. The benzodiazepines include diazepam, clorazepate, flurazepam, nitrazepam, lorazepam, triazolam, oxazepam, temazepam, chlordiazepoxide, clonazepam, and alprazolam. For the most part, all benzodiazepines act similarly to reduce anxiety. The difference is in their strength, how quickly they work, and their side effects. For example, clonazepam is long-lasting, takes up to 2 hours to work, and is generally taken two or three times a day. Alprazolam, on the other hand, works more quickly but wears off faster, thus requiring more doses. Increasing the number of doses makes it more likely a child will have to take the medication at school.

Benzodiazepines are usually used to treat anxiety disorders like separation anxiety, generalized anxiety disorder, and panic attacks in children and adolescents. They work by increasing the activity of a neurotransmitter known as GABA. GABA inhibits activity in the brain, so enhancing GABA activity leads to calmness.

Since this type of medication acts as a sedative, it can be expected that the most common short-term side effects are sleepiness and foggy thinking. Rarely, children will show lack of coordination (ataxia). There are some children who experience an opposite (paradoxical) reaction to sedation when they take a benzodiazapine. These children may become agitated or uninhibited when they take their medication. They may lose normal restraint of urges and impulses and may become talkative, agitated, silly, and more anxious. When this occurs, the family is usually told to wait a few hours until the medication leaves the child's system. Although this type of reaction can be extremely uncomfortable for the child and the child's caregivers, it usually does not signal a life-threatening problem. It is rare for children to become so agitated that they become a danger to themselves or others. When a child has had this type of reaction to a medication, they are usually prescribed a different medication.

Benzodiazpines can have adverse interactions when used with other drugs that have a sedative effect. There also can be adverse interactions with anticonvulsant medications. When benzodiazepines are abused, there is a risk that the individual will develop a dependence on the medication. Dependence can also occur at therapeutic doses with long-term use. This should provide a cautionary note to school personnel and parents about this aspect of these medications.

Another issue of concern is that benzodiazepines have a high potential for being sold or diverted to friends or family members. Physicians often will not provide the child with additional medication if this type of drug has been lost or has been used up before the end of the month, so it is important that medications be carefully monitored if they are stored at school. Each pill should be accounted for so that the child has enough of the medication needed. Rules regarding prescriptions of benzodiazepines are not as strict as those governing prescriptions of stimulants, but they are still carefully monitored by the DEA.

For some children, it is very important that they receive their benzodiazepine dose within a half hour of the scheduled time. Depending on the dosage and the type of medication, some children may begin to experience withdrawal symptoms if they do not receive their medication. Withdrawal symptoms vary depending on the potency and duration of the particular medicine. Dependence is most likely with high-potency, short-duration benzodiazepines like alprazolam, lorazepam, and triazolam, so withdrawal symptoms are worse with these medications.

In general, withdrawal symptoms include anxiety, irritability, insomnia, sweating, shakiness, fatigue, and gastrointestinal distress. More serious withdrawal effects include delirium and seizures. In the extreme, benzodiazepine withdrawal can result in death. It is important to ask families what they want the school to do if a dose is administered late or missed altogether.

Antihistamines

Antihistamines are usually used to treat allergies (e.g., diphenhydramine). These medications can cause sleepiness and relaxation and so are sometimes also used off-label to treat anxiety. They are not generally used over an extended period. Being quite sleepy can negatively affect a child's classroom performance, and teachers should alert a parent or physician if this becomes problematic.

Buspirone

Buspirone is an antianxiety medication that does not fit into any other class of medication. It is believed to affect levels of the neurotransmitters serotonin and dopamine in the brain. In addition to its usefulness in treating anxiety, buspirone is also helpful in treating irritability and aggression in children with developmental disabilities. Unlike benzodiazepines, which begin to take effect shortly after ingestion, this medication usually takes up to a month to reach its full level of effect. Buspirone is not as sedating as benzodiazepines. In addition, it has few side effects, including a very small likelihood of dependence. Side effects may include dizziness, nausea, headache, nervousness, lightheadedness, and excitement. If a dose of buspirone is missed, have the child take it as soon as it is remembered and alert the child's parents. Do not give the child two doses at the same time.

MOOD STABILIZERS

Mood stabilizers are used to treat mood swings, bipolar disorder, and aggression. Some mood stabilizers also are used to treat seizure disorders and in that role are called anticonvulsants or antiepileptics. An overview of the side effects commonly associated with several mood stabilizers is presented in Table 3.8.

Anticonvulsants

Anticonvulsants include carbamazepine, valproic acid, gabapentin, lamotrigine, topiramate, and tiagabine. Although they were developed for treatment of seizure disorders, they can be very useful in treating bipolar disorder, aggressive behavior, and severe mood

TABLE 3.8. Common Side Effects of Mood-Stabilizing Medications

Generic name	Trade name	Common side effects
Lithium salts	Lithobid, Lithonate, Lithotabs, Eskalith, Cibalith	Diarrhea, frequent urination, nausea, skin rashes, tremor, weight gain
Carbamazepine	Tegretol	Dizziness, drowsiness
Valproic acid	Valproate, Depakote	Cramps, stomach upset, diarrhea, indigestion, drowsiness, dizziness, lethargy (watch for liver problems)
Gabapentin	Neurontin	Fatigue, dizziness
Lamotrigine	Lamictal	Fatigue, rashes, dizziness, blurred or double vision
Topiramate	Topamax	Fatigue, dizziness, nervousness, tingling in extremities
Tiagabine	Gabitril	Fatigue, dizziness, unstable walking, associated with risk of seizures in patients without epilepsy treated off label

swings. Some children have abnormal electroencephalograms (brain wave measurements) but do not have a seizure disorder, and these medications may also be helpful in reducing behavior problems in this group of children. When a child is taking an anticonvulsant, it is important to monitor academic performance. Some anticonvulsants have been associated with impairments in cognitive performance.

It is possible to overdose on these medications. If a child misses a dose of an anticonvulsant, give it immediately and contact the child's parents to let them know what time the dose was received. The child's parents may need to adjust the times that the child receives later doses.

Lithium

Lithium salts are not anticonvulsants but are used to treat bipolar disorder in children and adults. Lithium is effective in treating bipolar disorder, especially acute mania. Lithium affects multiple neurotransmitters in the brain, including norepinephrine, dopamine, and serotonin. It is used to treat bipolar disorder, aggression, and very unstable moods. Lithium is considered to be a long-term medication and is often taken for 2 or more years. Lithium has a number of short-term side effects. The more common include nausea, vomiting, upset stomach, tremor, sleepiness, and weight gain. Lithium can make a child very thirsty, so bottled water and free trips to the drinking fountain and restroom should be allowed. Some children may report feeling dazed while taking this medication. Drowsiness and confusion can occur, which may impair the child's performance in school. Lithium can exacerbate acne. Hand tremor can occur, which is not dangerous but can be very distressing to the child. When possible, lithium should not be taken during pregnancy because of risk of harm to the developing fetus. It should be used with caution with adolescent girls who may be sexually active.

Lithium can accumulate to toxic levels that can damage the kidneys. Signs of lithium toxicity include difficulty walking or talking, vomiting, diarrhea, convulsions, and confusion. If these signs are observed in a child taking lithium, emergency medical personnel should be contacted immediately. Lithium requires blood level monitoring to ensure that an optimal dose is present in a child's system. Lithium should be given within a half hour of the scheduled time. Ask the family what they would like the school to do if the child's dose is late.

ANTIPSYCHOTICS

Antipsychotic medications also are sometimes called neuroleptics. There are two primary types of antipsychotic medications: traditional and atypical. The traditional antipsychotics include chlorpromazine, thioridazine, trifluoperazine, thiothixene, perphenazine, loxapine, haloperidol, fluphenazine, and pimozide. These medications affect the neurotransmitter dopamine. The atypical antipsychotics include clozapine, risperidone, olanzapine, and quetiapine fumarate. As with traditional antipsychotics, the atypical antipsychotics affect the neurotransmitter dopamine, but in a different way that is associated with fewer side effects. In addition, the atypical antipsychotics can also alleviate negative symptoms of psychosis, like social withdrawal and flat affect. Traditional antipsychotics tend to work best on the positive symptoms of psychosis such as hallucinations and delusions.

Antipsychotics are used to treat a wide range of symptoms and clinical problems (see Table 3.9 for a summary). They are effective in controlling psychotic symptoms like auditory hallucinations (hearing things that are not real), visual hallucinations (seeing things that are not there), and delusions (having odd beliefs). However, not all children who are prescribed an antipsychotic medication are suffering from psychosis. These medications are also often used in children without psychosis when other medications have not been successful. For example, they can be effective in reducing aggressive or self-injurious behavior, particularly in children with developmental disabilities. They also may help reduce explosiveness and stereotyped behaviors. They are useful in reducing tics such as those seen in Tourette's disorder.

TABLE 3.9. Symptoms Alleviated by Antipsychotic Medications

Auditory hallucinations
Visual hallucinations
Delusions and bizarre beliefs
Aggression
Self-injurious behavior
Social withdrawal
Overactivity
Stereotyped behavior seen in children with disabilities
Stuttering
Tic disorders (such as Tourette's disorder)

Side effects of the traditional and atypical antipsychotics are similar, but those of the atypical antipsychotics are often less severe. See Table 3.10 for a summary of side effects seen with some selected types of antipsychotic medications. A side effect frequently seen in this class of medication is sedation. A child may be sleepy and thinking may be foggy. Some children taking antipsychotics may have difficulty with learning and socialization. The effects of sedation on learning can be of particular concern when the child also has learning disability. Children on higher doses of medication seem to show more adverse side effects related to cognition and learning. Other side effects can include muscle spasms, muscle tightness, tremors, dry mouth, constipation, and blurred vision.

A serious side effect associated with long-term use of the traditional antipsychotics is known as tardive dyskinesia. Children who develop tardive dyskinesia display involuntary movements, particularly involuntary mouth and tongue movements. In some cases, the child may smack the lips as if chewing. In other cases, unusual tongue movements occur. Tardive dyskinesia is less likely to occur with the atypical antipsychotics, particularly with low doses. If symptoms of tardive dyskinesia are suspected, the child's parents should be alerted immediately and instructed to call the physician. These are serious side effects that can be difficult to reverse even when the medication is discontinued. See Table 3.11 for an overview of signs of tardive dyskinesia.

In very rare cases, children taking antipsychotic medications may experience an extremely serious, potentially fatal, reaction to the medication known as neuroleptic malignant syndrome. Signs can include confusion, fever, and sweating. A child who is experiencing these symptoms should be taken to the emergency room immediately. Make sure that emergency personnel know what medication the child is taking.

If a child misses a dose of an antipsychotic medication, give it as soon as it is remembered. Alert the child's parents so that they can make decisions about when to give their child the next dose. The child should not be given two doses at the same time.

TABLE 3.10. Common Side Effects of Antipsychotic Medications

Generic name	Trade name	Common side effects
Clozapine	Clozaril	Drowsiness, dizziness, low blood pressure, increased salivation, racing heartbeat, constipation
Haloperidol	Haldol	Akathisia, akinesia, sleepiness, low blood pressure, dry mouth, blurred vision, constipation, weight gain, difficulty urinating, stiffness
Thioridazine	Mellaril	Sleepiness, low blood pressure, dry mouth, blurred vision, constipation, weight gain, difficulty urinating, stiffness
Thiothixene	Navane	Sleepiness, low blood pressure, dry mouth, blurred vision, constipation, weight gain, difficulty urinating, stiffness
Olanzapine	Zyprexa	Drowsiness, dry mouth, dizziness, weakness, constipation, upset stomach, increased appetite, mild trembling
Risperidone	Risperdal	Sleepiness, low blood pressure, dry mouth, blurred vision, constipation, weight gain, difficulty urinating, nasal irritation and stuffiness, stiffness

TABLE 3.11. Signs of Tardive Dyskinesia

Tongue sticking or thrusting out of mouth
Grimacing facial expressions
Rapid eye blinking
Lip smacking, pursing, or puckering
Rapid movement of the arms or legs
Foot tapping or ankle movements
Shuffling while walking
Facial tics
Head movements to the back or side or head nodding

ANTIHYPERTENSIVES

Antihypertensive medications are traditionally used to treat high blood pressure in adults. In children, however, they are also effective in the treatment of tic disorders, ADHD, sleep disorders, and aggression. Antihypertensives include clonidine, guanfacine, and propranolol. The side effects associated with these medications are reviewed in Table 3.12.

Clonidine is used to treat ADHD, sleep disorders, tic disorders, and aggression. It is often the preferred treatment for Tourette's disorder because it simultaneously targets tics and symptoms of ADHD that often co-occur with Tourette's disorder. It is also used to treat children with developmental disabilities who are aggressive. Because it is sedating, it can be used to help children with sleep disturbances. This medication works quickly. However, because it is short acting, it must be taken multiple times during the day. This can lead to ups and downs in the child's behavior at school. Clonidine also can produce sedation, irritability, and depression. Guanfacine can be useful in treating ADHD, Tourette's disorder, and tics. Guanfacine can cause irritability, fatigue, and confusion at high doses, but these side effects may be less noticeable than those seen with clonidine. Propranolol is helpful with children with severe impulse control problems. Propranolol can result in nausea, vomiting, constipation or mild diarrhea, vivid dreams, depression, and (rarely) hallucinations. Propranolol also can cause slowing of the heart, reduction in blood pressure, and problems with breathing.

Once the medication is started, it must be given regularly and it should be discontinued only under a physician's supervision. This is because sudden withdrawal can cause high blood pressure.

TABLE 3.12. Common Side Effects of Antihypertensive Medications

Generic name	Trade name	Common side effects
Clonidine	Catapres	Sedation, depression, irritability, low blood pressure
Guanfacine	Tenex	Irritability, tiredness
Propranolol	Inderal	Nausea, vomiting, constipation, diarrhea, vivid dreams, depression, dizziness

If a child misses a dose of an antihypertensive medication, administer it as soon as it is remembered, as long as it is within an hour of the prescribed time. Do not give the child two doses at the same time. Alert the child's parents that the dose was received late.

SUMMARY

This chapter presents the complex world of psychopharmacology for children. There are several take-home messages. The first is that monitoring the effects of these medications on the delicate constitutions of children is crucial, since some very serious side effects can occur. The importance of monitoring leads to the second take-home message: Know about these medications. Use the tables in this book frequently to familiarize yourself with all aspects of these medications—including their effects and side effects and the symptoms they treat—so you can be a knowledgeable observer and effective member of the treatment team.

4

Child Psychiatric Disorders and Psychotropic Medications

The most common child psychiatric disorders are disruptive behavior disorders, anxiety disorders, mood disorders, tic disorders, developmental disabilities, psychotic disorders, and disorders of eating and elimination. Each category has specific diagnostic criteria from the latest edition of the *Diagnostic and Statistical Manual of Mental Disorders* (DSM-IV-TR; American Psychiatric Association, 2000). Each category has different symptoms, although there is also overlap of some symptoms among diagnoses. Some are easiest thought of as a spectrum that runs from no symptoms to the worst possible symptoms.

As you read through the following descriptions, you may recognize problems displayed by your students. Many children have symptoms of one or more disorders, but most do not meet the full criteria for diagnosis. Having symptoms but not meeting diagnostic criteria is a state referred to as subclinical. Being subclinical in terms of symptoms does not mean the child is not suffering or does not need some type of intervention.

Only a psychologist or physician can make the final determination about a child's diagnosis. However, observations and information provided by adults who work with the child are invaluable in making an accurate diagnosis. Symptoms that may not be obvious in a physician's or psychologist's office may be very problematic in other settings.

Many children who have significant behavioral or emotional problems may be accurately placed in more than one category of disorder. It is common for children to have two or more diagnoses at the same time. This is known as comorbidity. When a child has multiple diagnoses, the treatment team must decide whether to treat only one problem or multiple problems. This decision is usually based on the severity of each problem and on the nature of the comorbidity. There are three primary types of comorbidity:

1. Some disorders tend to occur simultaneously in certain children. For example, many children with Tourette's disorder also have significant symptoms of ADHD. On the other hand, most children with ADHD do not have Tourette's disorder. Having Tourette's

disorder puts a child at risk for having ADHD. In these cases, physicians often treat both disorders simultaneously. The child might receive one or more medications to treat symptoms of hyperactivity, inattention, and tics.

2. Sometimes, having one disorder can lead to the development of a second disorder. For example, some children with Asperger syndrome develop symptoms of depression. In some cases, depression may be related to the child's recognition of differentness from same-age peers and to feelings of social rejection. In these cases, the child's physician often chooses to treat the problem that is believed to be primary (the one that came first). In another example, if a child has obsessive–compulsive disorder (OCD) and depression, the doctor may choose to treat the obsessive–compulsive symptoms first with the hope that symptoms of depression will resolve when the child's other symptoms improve.

3. Some children have two or more disorders that are unrelated. Having one disorder does not protect the child from developing a second, unrelated problem. A child who has ADHD might develop separation anxiety or posttraumatic stress disorder (PTSD) that is unrelated to ADHD. In these cases, the child is usually treated for both disorders because treatment for one is not likely to heal the other.

ATTENTION PROBLEMS AND DISRUPTIVE BEHAVIOR DISORDERS

Attention problems and disruptive behavior disorders are grouped together because they frequently co-occur. Of course, not all children with ADHD suffer from behavior problems, often referred to as oppositional defiant disorder (ODD), and not all children with behavior problems have ADHD. However, approximately 50% of children with ADHD also have ODD. Some children with ODD later develop conduct disorder (CD), a very serious behavior disorder.

Attention-Deficit/Hyperactivity Disorder

There are three primary categories of ADHD. (See Table 4.1 for a summary.) The inattentive type of ADHD involves poor regulation of attention and includes symptoms like failing to pay close attention to assignments, making careless errors, being poorly organized, and being easily distracted. In the past, this disorder was called ADD because children with this disorder are not always hyperactive. In fact, they are sometimes slow or sluggish. This disorder is now called ADHD, predominantly inattentive type. ADHD, hyperactive–impulsive type, involves symptoms of both hyperactivity (i.e., being restless and fidgety) and impulsivity (i.e., interrupting and having difficulty waiting). The third type is ADHD, combined type, and involves symptoms of both the other two. This is the type most commonly encountered in classrooms.

Symptoms of ADHD tend to change and evolve as the child ages. Preschool children are more likely to be overly active and impulsive. In elementary school, children with ADHD tend to have symptoms like distractibility, low frustration tolerance, fidgeting, and

TABLE 4.1. Types of ADHD[1]

Predominantly inattentive	Predominantly hyperactive–impulsive	Combined
Makes careless errors.	Fidgety.	Symptoms from both columns.
Doesn't pay attention to detail.	Can't stay seated.	
Can't sustain attention, doesn't seem to listen.	Runs around.	
Doesn't finish work.	Always on the go.	
Can't organize.	Plays loudly.	
Avoids hard tasks.	Talks too much.	
Loses things.	Blurts out answers without raising hand.	
Easily distracted.	Can't wait for turn.	
Forgetful.	Interrupts others.	

[1]Other diagnostic criteria for ADHD include symptoms prior to the age of 7 years for a duration of at least 6 months, documentation indicating that the symptoms occur in at least 2 places (e.g., school, home), and evidence of functional impairment (e.g., academic failure, poor peer relationships).

difficulty with sustained attention. These symptoms typically are apparent at home, at school, and in peer interactions. Although symptoms of hyperactivity and inattention decrease over time, children with ADHD are likely to struggle with the disorder in adolescence and adulthood. As adults, they may be disorganized, forget to pay bills, make impulsive decisions, or have difficulty completing work assignments.

Although many children with ADHD do not have other behavioral or emotional problems, some children have other difficulties that may also need treatment. About half of all children with ADHD also have ODD and about 1 in 10 have CD. Learning problems are also common.

Table 4.2 is a summary of some of the medications commonly prescribed for children with ADHD. Stimulants are the most widely researched and prescribed medications in child psychiatry and are often used in the treatment of ADHD. Stimulants work because they stimulate the areas of the brain that control attention and regulate behavior. These medications have an excellent safety record and reliable results.

The beneficial effects of stimulants for the treatment of symptoms of ADHD are well documented. Stimulants are often used as a first option for children with ADHD for several reasons.

1. One benefit of using stimulant medications is that doses can be missed without significant harm. Parents may be able to give the child stimulants only on school days and avoid use of the medication during the summer or on weekends.
2. Unlike other medications that may take several weeks to start working, stimulants usually start working as soon as they enter the child's system. Therefore, if the medication is going to work, the child should quickly show decreased activity levels, better concentration, and better control of behavior. If these effects are not noticeable within an hour after taking the medication, the child may not be receiv-

ing the correct dose or the medication may not be working. This allows physicians to make adjustments quickly when medications are not effective.

3. As with any medication, stimulants can have negative side effects. These medications work quickly and leave the body quickly. If a negative side effect is observed, the child can simply stop taking the medication and the negative side effects will wear off within 3 to 8 hours.

4. Some of the older stimulants such as Ritalin have been used for more than 30 years and are considered to be extremely safe.

A child who is prescribed a stimulant medication may initially take a small dose of the medication, and then the dose is increased over a period of several weeks until the optimal dose is achieved. In some cases, children may not respond well to one stimulant medication and a different one will be prescribed. Examples of poor response to medication include negative side effects and symptoms not improving. In the past, one concern with stimulants was that children usually needed to take one dose in the morning before school and one dose at school during lunch. There are now sustained-release stimulant medications that are taken once per day.

TABLE 4.2. Medications for ADHD

Generic (trade) name	Class	Notes
Amphetamine (Adderall)	Stimulant	Can cause appetite suppression, insomnia, dizziness, gastrointestinal problems and irritability; watch for tics.
Dextroamphetamine (Dexedrine)	Stimulant	Can cause appetite suppression, insomnia, dizziness, gastrointestinal problems and irritability; watch for tics
Methylphenidate (Concerta, Metadate, Ritalin)	Stimulant	Can cause appetite suppression, insomnia, dizziness, gastrointestinal problems and irritability; watch for tics.
Atomoxetine HCL (Strattera)	—	Can cause nausea, appetite suppression, dizziness, fatigue, mood swings.
Bupropion (Wellbutrin)	Atypical antidepressant	Insomnia, dizziness, constipation, irritability, decreased appetite; watch for tics.
Desipramine (Norpramin)	TCA	Can cause cardiac complications leading to death; not often recommended by physicians.
Nortriptyline (Aventyl, Pamelor)	TCA	Can cause dry mouth, constipation, nausea, blurred vision, sedation, stomach upset, nightmares; overdose risk.
Imipramine (Tofranil)	TCA	Can cause dry mouth, constipation, nausea, blurred vision, sedation, stomach upset, nightmares; overdose risk.
Clonidine (Catapres)	Antihypertensive	Can cause sedation, hypotension, irritability, and depression.
Guanfacine (Tenex)	Antihypertensive	Can cause dry mouth, drowsiness, dizziness, constipation, headache, upset stomach.

The use of stimulant medications has dramatically increased in the past two decades. It has been argued that this rise reflects both an overreliance on medication management of ADHD and overdiagnosis of the disorder in general. Others have argued that stimulant medication is actually underused in the management of children with ADHD and that the increase in use is related to better recognition of the disorder.

When stimulants are ineffective or negative side effects from treatment are unacceptable, antidepressant medications are sometimes used to treat ADHD (Reiff & Tippins, 2004). In contrast to stimulants, the effects of antidepressant medications often take at least 4 weeks to evaluate. One benefit of antidepressants is that the effects are consistent across the day. Stimulants wear off by homework or dinner time, but antidepressants remain at stable levels as long as the child continues to take the medications daily. Additionally, because the timing of the dose is less precise, these medications can usually be given at home and not at school. Because antidepressants are not controlled substances, refills can be phoned in by the child's physician, giving parents more leeway. In contrast to stimulants, it is not appropriate to skip a dose of antidepressant medications.

Traditional antidepressant medications that are used to treat ADHD include tricylic antidepressants such as desipramine, imipramine, and nortriptyline (Reiff & Tippins, 2004). Wellbutrin, an atypical antidepressant, is also effective in treating ADHD. Another medication in this class now used to treat ADHD is atomoxetine HCL. While this medication was previously developed as an antidepressant, it is now used to treat ADHD. Its effects in the brain are similar to these of an antidepressant. It is a selective norepinephrine reuptake inhibitor originally designed specifically to treat depression in adults.

Some children with ADHD benefit from treatment with the antihypertensive medications such as clonidine and guanfacine. These medications may be particularly useful for children with ADHD who are agitated or aggressive. The following is an example.

> Jason is 16 years old and is just beginning his junior year in high school. He was diagnosed with ADHD in the second grade and took medication for the management of ADHD through the seventh grade. Although he is no longer overly active, his parents and teachers continue to have concerns about his academic performance. He seems to have special difficulty planning in advance for semester-long projects and comprehensive final exams. Although he is bright and does well on exams, he often receives mediocre semester grades because of missing homework assignments. He takes poor notes during class because he is easily distracted. In addition to these concerns, Jason has received a speeding ticket and has been involved in two fender benders since receiving his license only 4 months ago. His mother is starting to have serious concerns about her son's ability to complete college without her assistance.

There is no medication that will teach Jason time-management skills. These skills need to be specifically taught, and Jason will probably always require assistance in planning long-term projects. It is important that his parents help him access services for students with disabilities when he gets to college. However, now that Jason is driving, his impulsivity is a serious concern. He has already demonstrated poor decision-making while driving. It may make sense for Jason to resume the stimulant medication that worked for him when he was a child. This may have the added benefit of helping him to be less distractible during class lectures. One concern about the use of stimulant medications with teenagers is the possibility that the medication can be sold for improper use. If this is a concern, nonstimulant medication treatment can be prescribed or his parents can control administration of the medication.

Oppositional Defiant Disorder

ODD is a pattern of defiant behavior that persists over time and settings. Children with ODD frequently argue with adults, lose their tempers, and defy rules. They may be irritable and easily annoyed. ODD is often diagnosed during early elementary school, around age 6. However, in most cases, behavior problems like tantrums, stubbornness, and defiance can be traced back to as early as age 3. In most cases, the treatment of choice for ODD is behavior therapy. However, when ODD occurs with ADHD, treatment of ADHD symptoms can sometimes improve symptoms of ODD. Additionally, it is important to determine whether the child truly has ODD or whether irritable, negative behaviors are masking an underlying depression that may require both behavior therapy and medication.

Conduct Disorder

CD involves very serious behavior problems that violate the rights of others. Behaviors may include aggression, property destruction, cruelty to people or animals, fire setting, stealing, running away, or truancy. These behaviors typically occur in multiple settings. There is no medication to treat CD; individual and family behavior therapy are usually recommended. However, many children in this group are also diagnosed with other disorders like ADHD or mood disorders. In these cases, medication may be prescribed to manage symptoms of the second disorder, but medication management must be approached very carefully. Adolescents with CD are at high risk for illegal diversion of medications.

ANXIETY DISORDERS

Almost everyone has times when they feel anxious or nervous. Symptoms of anxiety are often observed in children who do not have psychiatric problems. For example, most infants between 6 and 18 months of age become distressed when separated from their primary caregiver. Starting at about 10 months of age, most babies also begin to be fearful of strangers. Preschool children are often afraid of the dark. School-aged children may worry about doing well in school. Many adolescents have anxiety related to social performance and social evaluation. These somewhat common symptoms of anxiety may become abnormal when they last for a long time or interfere with the child's quality of life. Anxiety problems can be distressing for the child and the child's social circle. Anxious children may have chronic stomachaches, headaches, and other physical problems. Their school performance may suffer if they resist attending school, fail to ask for clarification or assistance, or refuse to perform required academic activities (e.g., giving a class presentation). Some anxious children also perform poorly on tests even when they have studied for the exam and know the information.

Experts believe that most anxiety disorders are the result of both environmental and genetic factors. Some babies just seem to be born with very shy temperaments and tend to be very cautious in exploring their surroundings. These babies are more likely to develop problems with anxiety that rise to a clinical level later in childhood or adulthood. Additionally, many anxious children have anxious parents. The parents pass on their genetic predisposition toward anxiety and may also model and reinforce anxious behavior in their children.

In this section, we discuss seven disorders that are related to anxiety. These include separation anxiety disorder, generalized anxiety disorder (GAD), panic disorder, selective mutism, phobias, OCD, and PTSD. (See Table 4.3 for a summary.)

New research suggests that childhood anxiety disorders are more prevalent than previously believed and that these disorders persist over time. Childhood anxiety disorders can often be treated with behavioral, cognitive-behavioral, and psychosocial interventions. Very few double-blind studies (experiments where neither the experimenter nor the participants know if the participant is taking actual medication or a placebo) have been conducted to explore the efficacy of medications for childhood anxiety problems. Unfortunately, it is becoming increasingly common for children with these disorders to be treated with medication alone.

It is usually recommended that medication be used only with children who have not responded to other therapies for anxiety or that medication be used only in conjunction with other therapies. In addition, medication for anxiety is usually used only for a short time and is discontinued once symptoms improve. Anxious children are often given medication for vague problems (e.g., school refusal, irritability, headaches and stomachaches) that would be treated more effectively with other therapies. Improvement is difficult to assess in gauging treatment effectiveness. As a result, symptom reduction is not always used as a guideline for decision making.

TABLE 4.3. Types of Anxiety Disorders

Disorder	Major symptoms
Separation anxiety disorder	Anxiety related to separation from the parent or the home
Generalized anxiety disorder (GAD)	Excessive worry about typical life events and activities
Panic disorder	Recurrent and unexpected bouts of sudden and intense fear
Selective mutism	Failure to speak in specific social situations (e.g., failure to speak at school)
Phobias	Excessive fear of a specific object or situation
Obsessive–compulsive disorder (OCD)	Intrusive, distressing thoughts or repetitive behaviors
Posttraumatic stress disorder (PTSD)	Symptoms of intense distress or emotional numbing following exposure to a life-threatening event

Table 4.4 provides an overview of medications used in treating children with anxiety disorders. One type of medication that is used to treat anxiety disorders is benzodiazepines, which includes diazepam and clonazepam. Separation anxiety disorder, GAD, and panic disorder can be treated with clonazepam, which can decrease the frequency of panic attacks and decrease symptoms of anxiety. Side effects can include drowsiness, clumsiness (poor coordination or ataxia), and dizziness. Conversely, some people experience a paradoxical (opposite) reaction when taking benzodiazepines and become very nervous and agitated. A paradoxical reaction is not dangerous but can be very distressing to the child. The symptoms will disappear when the medication leaves the child's system, usually within a few hours.

Certain antidepressants can also be effective in treating anxiety disorders. Clomipramine is a TCA that has been documented in double-blind studies to decrease symptoms of

TABLE 4.4. Medications for the Management of Anxiety Disorders in Children

Generic (trade) name	Class	Notes and side effects
Clonidine (Catapres)	Antihypertensive	Effective in treating PTSD; can cause sedation, hypotension, irritability, and depression.
Propranolol (Inderal)	Antihypertensive	Effective in treating PTSD; can cause reduced blood pressure, drowsiness, and insomnia.
Buspirone (Buspar)	Atypical antianxiety	Effective in treating GAD, social phobia, panic disorder, separation anxiety disorder; can cause dizziness, confusion, disinhibition and drowsiness.
Clonazepam (Klonopin)	Benzodiazepine	Effective in treating GAD, panic disorder, separation anxiety; can cause drowsiness, ataxia, dizziness; watch for agitation or disinhibition (paradoxical reaction).
Lorazepam (Ativan)	Benzodiazepine	Can cause drowsiness, ataxia, dizziness; watch for agitation or disinhibition (paradoxical reaction).
Fluoxetine (Prozac)	SSRI	Effective in treating OCD, panic, separation anxiety; can cause restlessness, nausea, insomnia, fatigue, decreased appetite, tremors, disinhibition, agitation, stomach upset, headaches.
Sertraline (Zoloft)	SSRI	Effective in treating OCD, panic, separation anxiety; can cause restlessness, nausea, insomnia, fatigue, decreased appetite, tremors, disinhibition, agitation, stomach upset, headaches.
Fluvoxamine (Luvox)	SSRI	Effective in treating OCD, panic, separation anxiety; can cause restlessness, nausea, insomnia, fatigue, decreased appetite, tremors, disinhibition, agitation, stomach upset, headaches.
Paroxetine (Paxil)	SSRI	Effective in treating OCD, panic, separation anxiety; can cause restlessness, nausea, insomnia, fatigue, decreased appetite, tremors, disinhibition, agitation, stomach upset, headaches.
Clomipramine (Anafranil)	TCA	Effective in treating OCD; watch for seizures with prolonged use and high doses; can cause dry mouth, constipation, nausea, blurred vision, sedation, stomach upset, nightmares, fatigue; overdose risk.

OCD in children. Children being treated with clomipramine require monitoring of heart and liver functioning. There is a risk of seizure if children are treated with the medication for more than 1 year. Other common side effects include drowsiness, dizziness, tremors, headaches, and dry mouth. Although both desipramine and imipramine have been shown to be somewhat effective in treating anxious children, the risk of death due to cardiac complications makes these medications more risky choices.

More recently, SSRI antidepressants have gained popularity for use with anxious children. Fluoxetine has been used successfully to treat OCD, separation anxiety disorder, and social phobia. Sertraline, paroxetine, and fluvoxamine treat OCD. SSRI antidepressants may be used when a child with PTSD also suffers from depression. Again, these are off-label uses that must be monitored carefully. Side effects can include tiredness, insomnia, restlessness, and nausea.

Buspirone, a medication used to manage anxiety in adults, is also effective in the treatment of GAD in children. Antihypertensives have been used to treat anxiety disorders, particularly PTSD, in children. Clonidine and propranolol have been used to treat PTSD symptoms of overarousal.

Separation Anxiety Disorder

Separation anxiety disorder is one of the most common childhood problems. Age-appropriate separation anxiety starts as early as 6 months and may last as long as 2 years. Infants and toddlers may become very upset when they are left with grandparents or babysitters, even when these caregivers are well known to the child. However, when these same symptoms persist into early school age, the child may be suffering from separation anxiety disorder. Children with this disorder are very anxious about being away from home or being separated from their primary caretaker. They may worry frequently about the safety of their caretaker. They may also refuse to go to school, go to sleep, or stay home without their primary caregiver. Children with separation anxiety may also have problems like nightmares, headaches, and stomachaches that become worse when separation is anticipated.

Generalized Anxiety Disorder

Children with GAD worry excessively about normal, everyday life events. Unlike children with OCD, who may worry about a bizarre or unlikely outcome (such as being severely contaminated through contact with a toilet seat), children with GAD worry excessively about such everyday concerns as performing well on a test, pleasing their parents, or being able to complete responsibilities. Of course, it is not unusual for children (and adults) to worry about routine life events. However, the child with GAD may be unable to complete homework or to concentrate in school because of the inability to stop worrying. The child may also have difficulty initiating or completing assignments because of anxiety. Children with GAD may have physical symptoms like headaches or stomachaches and may habitually stay home sick on the day of a big test.

Panic Disorder

Panic disorder often develops during adolescence, with the peak age of onset occurring between 15 and 19 years of age. Children and adolescents with panic disorder experience recurrent panic symptoms that are severe enough to warrant the word "attack" to describe them. These symptoms typically develop without warning and include very intense feelings of fear and symptoms like sweating, shaking, shortness of breath, nausea, dizziness, a racing heart, and chest pain. The child or adolescent may have fears of going crazy or dying. Panic attacks are extremely distressing to the individual, but for many people, the fear of panic attacks can be more debilitating than the actual attacks themselves. People with panic disorder typically live with a persistent fear of experiencing another attack. In some cases, this fear may be so marked that the child may refuse to leave the house (agoraphobia). In these cases, the child may be particularly resistant to going places where it may be difficult to leave during a panic attack (e.g., a bus, a concert, a crowded mall). There is a great deal of evidence to suggest that panic disorder is genetic.

Selective Mutism

Selective mutism is not necessarily an anxiety-related disorder, although it is often grouped with the anxiety disorders. Children with selective mutism fail to use language in certain situations, usually at school or in public. Many children with selective mutism speak freely at home. Unlike children with mental retardation or children with speech delays, children with selective mutism are capable of talking and usually talk freely in one or more situations. Some children may talk only to immediate family members. Selective mutism is usually not diagnosed when the child refuses to speak because of a speech impediment and is embarrassed or afraid that the listener will not understand. Selectively mute children are usually shy, nervous, and fearful.

> Six-year-old Maggie is a first grader in Ms. Page's class. She usually responds to questions with a brief yes-or-no nod. On rare occasions she will whisper answers that are so quiet, Ms. Page can barely hear her. When asked a direct question requiring more than a nod, Maggie usually sucks on her fingers and stares blankly at Ms. Page. During the first parent conference, Ms. Page was shocked to hear Maggie's mother describe her behavior at home as loud, boisterous, and even bossy with her younger siblings.

It is very important that Maggie's selective mutism be treated as quickly as possible. There are excellent behavior therapy approaches to the treatment of this problem. Maggie might also be helped by an SSRI or an anxiolytic medication while she works through the initial phases of psychological intervention.

Phobias

A phobia occurs when a child has an excessive fear of something like heights, small spaces, or spiders. A specific phobia is diagnosed when the child has a fear of a specific object or situation. Common phobias are fear of the dark, fear of spiders, and fear of needles. A social phobia is diagnosed when the child is afraid of being embarrassed in a social situation. Class presentations can be so difficult for children with social phobia that they may refuse to go to school or to participate when presentations are scheduled. Likewise, even seemingly easy responsibilities such as saying hello to a new classmate or asking for help in class can be almost impossible for a child with social phobia.

It can be difficult to differentiate between normal childhood fears and a true phobia. Many young children are fearful of strangers, animals, or monsters. Although these childhood fears can be very distressing to the child and family, their duration is usually short. A phobia is diagnosed when the fear persists over time and interferes with the child's daily life. For example, an 8-year-old who refuses to go outside or to watch TV because a snake might appear may have a phobia. On the other hand, a 3-year-old who avoids going to bed at night because she is afraid of the dark probably does not have a phobia.

Some phobias develop after the child has been exposed to a frightening event, such as watching a sibling get bitten by a bee. Family members may inadvertently reinforce other phobias. An example of this is a child who receives special time with mom at bedtime because of a fear of monsters. Humans in general seem to be biologically predisposed to develop phobias to certain dangers like snakes and spiders. Some scientists believe that these fears kept our ancestors safe by keeping them from having contact with things that could hurt them.

Obsessive–Compulsive Disorder

OCD often involves intrusive thoughts or images (obsessions) or impulses (compulsions). For example, a child may have obsessive fears of contamination or of death. The child may engage in repetitive behaviors or mental acts in an attempt to reduce the stress felt from the thoughts. Compulsive acts may include repetitive hand washing (often related to contamination obsessions), ritualistic touching of objects, or counting. Some children with OCD have intrusive thoughts that are upsetting to them, often with violent or sexual images. Some children may feel anxious when items are not arranged in a symmetrical manner or when a pencil is not perfectly sharp. OCD often develops during childhood or adolescence. Although no single gene for the disorder has been identified, research suggests that children with this disorder are born with biological risk factors that are exacerbated by stress. There are excellent psychotherapeutic treatments for OCD. The behavioral approach of exposure plus response prevention is an effective treatment. In this therapy, the child is placed in a situation where the stimulus occurs and then any response to that stimulus (such as counting, for instance) is prevented. Medications may be prescribed in conjunction with behavioral psychotherapy

Allie is an 11-year-old who is in the sixth grade. At the beginning of the school year, Allie was doing well in school. She completed her work carefully and on time and usually received A's on tests. For the last few months, Allie's performance has fallen off dramatically. She seems to have trouble finishing her work. It can take her 2 hours to complete a short quiz that takes the other students less than half an hour. She reviews her answers over and over and often erases words that aren't written perfectly. Most of her papers are returned with holes in them because she has erased the answers so many times. She is constantly arranging and rearranging her materials on her desk so that they are "just so." Her mother has complained that she is receiving 6 hours per night of homework. Her teacher has reported that 1 hour of homework has been assigned.

Allie's behaviors may be consistent with a diagnosis of OCD. Children with OCD may doubt that they have completed an assignment correctly, so they may check it over and over. Of course, no matter how many times Allie checks it, she will continue to have doubting feelings. She may have a difficult time getting started on work because things must be arranged in a certain way (her pencils must be sharpened in a certain manner and books must be aligned) or certain mental rituals must be accomplished (counting in a specific way or waiting for a sign) before work can begin. Many children with compulsive behaviors will admit to having intrusive and unwanted thoughts as well. It is important that Allie receive a full evaluation. If she does have OCD, the best treatment is the behavioral treatment of exposure plus response prevention. Allie may also benefit from treatment with an antidepressant.

Posttraumatic Stress Disorder

PTSD is characterized by the development of significant psychological problems following exposure to a life-threatening event such as a car accident, an assault, or a natural disaster. Some children experience PTSD after hearing about a loved one being exposed to a life-threatening event. Following the traumatic incident, the child may feel as if the event is happening all over again (reexperiencing symptoms), have bad dreams about the incident, suddenly replay the event (flashbacks), or have distressing thoughts that the trauma will intrude unexpectedly. The child might also experience distress when exposed to reminders of the trauma. For example, a child who has been in a very serious car accident may become upset when riding in a car. Children with PTSD may also become emotionally numb and try to avoid thinking or talking about the trauma. They may seem to be detached from family and friends. They might show signs of increased stress, sleeping difficulties, irritability, or difficulty concentrating.

There are excellent psychotherapies to help children who have suffered a traumatic event, but no medication specifically treats PTSD. However, in addition to psychotherapy, medication is sometimes prescribed to help with problematic symptoms that interfere with or slow the child's progress in therapy. Sleep medications, for example, may be prescribed for a child who is too anxious or frightened to sleep.

MOOD DISORDERS

We all have times when we are blue or sad. However, when a child loses interest in activities that used to be enjoyable and is gloomy and down for days or weeks at a time, a mood disorder such as depression may be present. Mood disorders also include symptoms opposite from depression, like extreme laughter and happiness, excessive irritability, and hyperwakefulness. These are symptoms of mania and are sometimes associated with bipolar disorder. Bipolar simply means moods that are at the two extremes of a continuum (or pole) of mood. The two major types of mood disorders are depressive disorders (including dysthymia) and bipolar disorders.

Depressive Disorders

Depression in children can be more difficult to recognize than depression in adults. Adults with depression are likely to report feelings of sadness; children with depression are more likely to show symptoms like chronic irritability, poor energy, disturbed sleep patterns, and changes in appetite. Physical complaints such as vague aches and pains, stomachaches, and headaches are common. They may describe themselves as bored. Children with depression may also begin to perform poorly in school. Symptoms like temper tantrums, behavior problems, and difficulty with peers can also signal depression in children.

Some children may experience a major depressive episode, which lasts at least 2 weeks and is marked by symptoms of sadness, irritability, or loss of interest in things the child used to enjoy. A child with major depression may have difficulty concentrating in school or making decisions. There may be weight loss or gain for no apparent reason. Some children with depression have difficulty falling asleep or staying asleep while others seem to sleep all the time. Some depressed children can become agitated and restless. Others have poor energy and move slowly and sluggishly. The child may think or talk about death or suicide.

Another depressive disorder sometimes observed in children is called dysthymic disorder, and it is somewhat of a low-grade depression. Children with dysthymia have a chronically depressed or irritable mood that lasts for more than a year. Like children with depression, they may have problems with their appetite, sleep schedule, and energy level. They may also report that they feel worthless or may show signs of poor self-esteem. They may have difficulty concentrating in class or making decisions.

It can be difficult to distinguish between day-to-day mood variations and a true problem with depression. Some children and adolescents become extremely upset over small mishaps or minor incidents. These children may simply have a temperament that is especially sensitive or reactive. Similarly, it is normal for a child or adolescent to feel sad following the death of a loved one. On the other hand, if a child stays upset for a prolonged period following an upsetting incident, this may be a sign of depression.

Table 4.5 provides an overview of medications used to treat mood disorders in children. Although many antidepressant medications (particularly SSRIs and TCAs) have excellent outcomes with adults, their effectiveness with children is still being researched and is not yet fully understood. At this point, medications are often reserved for use when other treatments have not been effective or when the child's depression is very severe. Further, there have been some reports of suicidality in children taking SSRI medications. At this writing, this relationship is being researched, and the FDA is requiring black box warnings regarding suicide to be placed on the package information of all SSRI antidepressants except Prozac. Regardless of the type of treatment a child is receiving, suicidality

TABLE 4.5. Medications for the Management of Mood Disorders in Children

Generic (trade) name	Class	Indicated use	Side effects
Carbamezepine (Tegretol)	Antiepileptic	Mania	Dizziness, drowsiness, nausea, blurred vision; watch for rash; need to monitor white blood cell count.
Valproic acid (Depakote)	Antiepileptic	Mania	Nausea, vomiting, indigestion, sedation, dizziness, weight gain, appetite suppression; requires blood level monitoring; watch for pancreatic swelling.
Clozapine (Clozaril)	Atypical antipsychotic	Bipolar symptoms	Cognitive sedation, extrapyramidal effects.
Risperidone (Risperdal)	Atypical antipsychotic	Mania	Cognitive sedation, extrapyramidal effects.
Lithium (Eskalith, Lithane, Lithobid, Lithonate)	Mood stabilizer	Mania	Can cause diarrhea, nausea, tremor, drowsiness, memory impairment; requires blood level monitoring; monitor for toxicity.
Fluoxetine (Prozac)	SSRI	Depression	Can cause restlessness, nausea, insomnia, fatigue, decreased appetite, tremors, disinhibition, agitation, stomach upset, headaches.
Fluvoxamine (Luvox)	SSRI	Depression	Can cause restlessness, nausea, insomnia, fatigue, decreased appetite, tremors, disinhibition, agitation, stomach upset, headaches.
Paroxetine (Paxil)	SSRI	Depression	Can cause restlessness, nausea, insomnia, fatigue, decreased appetite, tremors, disinhibition, agitation, stomach upset, headaches.
Sertraline (Zoloft)	SSRI	Depression	Can cause restlessness, nausea, insomnia, fatigue, decreased appetite, tremors, disinhibition, agitation, stomach upset, headaches.
Citalopram (Celexa)	SSRI	Depression	Can cause restlessness, nausea, insomnia, fatigue, decreased appetite, tremors, disinhibition, agitation, stomach upset, headaches.
Clomipramine (Anafranil)	TCA	Depression	Risk of seizure onset with prolonged use and high dosage; can cause dry mouth, constipation, nausea, blurred vision, sedation, stomach upset, nightmares; overdose risk.

is always a concern when children are depressed. For this reason, careful monitoring of depressed children is always necessary.

Bipolar Disorder

Physicians used to believe that bipolar disorder occurred only in adolescents and adults. Recently, however, there has been increased understanding of bipolar disorder in children. Bipolar disorder is characterized by periods of mania (manic episodes) or mild mania (hypomanic episodes) generally alternating with depression. Manic episodes involve at least a weeklong period where the child has an abnormally elevated or irritable mood. This mood represents a marked change from the child's normal behavior. The child may act indestructible and may engage in dangerous behaviors. A child may seem rested after having little or no sleep or might talk excessively or report thoughts that are racing. Behavior may be agitated, restless, or very active. It may be extremely difficult to get the child's attention. Children who have one or more manic episodes are diagnosed with bipolar I disorder. These children may also be at risk for the development of depression. However, not all children with bipolar I disorder have depressive episodes.

A hypomanic episode is similar to a manic episode but lasts for a shorter period and has less severe symptoms. Children who have one or more hypomanic episodes plus one or more depressive episodes are diagnosed with bipolar II disorder.

There is also evidence that some children with bipolar disorder do not have the discrete mood episodes (mania and depression) discussed above. Instead, they may rapidly cycle from depression to mania in a period of hours or days. Some children may also experience symptoms of mania and depression at the same time.

Unlike children with depression, who are often successfully treated with psychotherapy, children with bipolar disorder almost always require treatment with medication. The medications used for bipolar disorder include lithium and mood stabilizers (antiepileptic medications). Lithium carbonate is the classic treatment for bipolar disorder. This medication accumulates in the child's bloodstream, so frequent monitoring of blood levels is necessary to ensure the child is receiving the optimal dose and to avoid side effects and toxic reactions. The side effects of lithium can make this medication difficult for some children to tolerate even when it is effective in managing symptoms. Side effects can include nausea, fatigue, tremors, and cognitive problems. Many children taking lithium will be extremely thirsty. They may need to keep a water bottle by their desk or they may need permission to make unlimited trips to the drinking fountain. Some children will also experience significant weight gain and exacerbation of acne. Dangerous toxic reactions can be signaled by symptoms such as vomiting, diarrhea, tremors, or convulsions. Pregnant teenagers should not take lithium because this medication can damage the developing baby.

Antiepileptic medications are often used as mood stabilizers for children with bipolar disorder. For example, carbamazepine and valproic acid may be used to treat children with bipolar disorder even when seizures are not present. Like lithium, blood level monitoring is necessary with these medications. Side effects can include fatigue, nausea, dizziness, weight gain, appetite loss, and blurry vision. Children taking carbamazepine should also be monitored for the development of a rash that affects the hands and mouth. Other antiepileptic medications used to manage mood symptoms include gabapentin, lamotrigine, oxcarbazepine, tiagabine, and topiramate.

Bipolar disorder is usually complicated. Children with bipolar disorder may also suffer from ADHD, anxiety, or psychosis. Children with ADHD and bipolar disorder will likely require treatment for both disorders (i.e., a stimulant and a mood stabilizer). Similarly, when the child also has psychotic symptoms such as hallucinations or bizarre thoughts, an antipsychotic may also be needed. In some complex cases, children with bipolar disorder may require more than two medications to manage symptoms effectively.

Greg is a 10-year-old boy who is in the fourth grade. His teacher knows that he has ADHD and is on medication for this problem. She has made a number of accommodations to help him focus and stay organized. However, his behavior continues to be very problematic. He is extremely irritable and tends to overreact to even small conflicts in the classroom. A couple of weeks ago, Greg's behavior improved and, although he was still irritable, he was quiet and sedate. More recently, he has become increasingly agitated, loud, and disruptive in class. A day rarely passes that Greg doesn't cry or end up in a yelling match with another child. It seems as though the smallest event can send him from perfectly calm to near hysteria. His teacher is starting to wonder if his problems extend beyond ADHD.

Greg's behavior problems are not typical of a child with simple ADHD and may reflect an underlying mood disorder. It would be helpful for Greg's teacher to document her observations for several weeks so that Greg's parents and doctors can get a better idea of the types of problems he is having. Irritability is a common symptom of childhood depression. On the other hand, Greg's mood swings may suggest pediatric bipolar disorder. It will be important to find out whether Greg's variations in mood have anything to do with other events in his life.

TIC DISORDERS

A tic is a recurrent movement or vocalization. Motor tics can be simple (e.g., eye blinking, grimacing, and coughing) or complex (e.g., jumping, touching, and smelling). Simple motor tics are relatively common in young children and most children are unaware that they are even occurring. Complex motor tics last longer and may be more purposeful (e.g., smelling an object). Some children may also have self-injurious tics like slapping, hitting, or biting themselves. Vocal tics, which are similar to motor tics, can also be simple (e.g., grunting, barking) or complex (e.g., repeating words and phrases).

Most tic disorders begin before age 10. They tend to emerge first between ages 6 and 7, and many disappear or become markedly less severe by age 18. Motor tics such as eye blinking usually emerge first. Vocal tics usually emerge several years later. Tic disorders are often worst during preadolescence, between 8 and 12 years of age.

Somewhere between 10 and 20% of children will experience a transient tic at some time during childhood. However, a tic disorder is diagnosed when the tic persists over time. There are several categories of tic disorders, with the most severe being Tourette's disorder (TD). Children with TD have chronic motor and vocal tics. Children with TD are at risk for ADHD and OCD.

Psychopharmacological interventions are the most common treatments for patients with TD, and tics can generally be controlled with proper medication in about 80% of cases. Table 4.6 provides an overview of medications used to treat tic disorders in children. Medications previously used to control hypertension are often the first line of treatment for TD. The side effects of these medications are generally mild, and they also may improve symptoms of ADHD that are often comborbid with TD. These medications include guanfacine and clonidine. A failed trial of an antihypertensive is often followed by a low dose of a neuroleptic medication such as risperidone or haloperidol. The atypical antipsychotics (e.g., risperidone, olanzapine, ziprasidone, and quetiapine) are usually used before the traditional antipsychotics (e.g., haloperidol, pimozide) because they have fewer

TABLE 4.6. Medications for the Management of Tic Disorders in Children

Generic (trade) name	Class	Side effects
Clonidine (Catapres)	Antihypertensive	Can cause sedation, hypotension, irritability, and depression; can reduce symptoms of ADHD as well as tics.
Guanfacine (Tenex)	Antihypertensive	Can cause hypotension and sedation; reduces symptoms of ADHD as well as tics.
Haloperidol (Haldol)	Antipsychotic	Can cause sedation, weight gain, cognitive blunting, decreased seizure threshold; must monitor for movement disorders.
Pimozide (Orap)	Antipsychotic	Can cause sedation, weight gain, cognitive blunting, decreased seizure threshold; must monitor for movement disorders.
Risperidone (Risperdal)	Atypical antipsychotic	Can cause sedation, weight gain, cognitive blunting, decreased seizure threshold; must monitor for movement disorders.
Olanzapine (Zyprexa)	Atypical antipsychotic	Can cause sedation, weight gain, cognitive blunting, decreased seizure threshold; must monitor for movement disorders.

and less severe side effects. Other treatments are used when these agents are not successful or when adverse side effects are intolerable.

Because some children with TD also suffer from significant ADHD, the stimulant medications used to treat ADHD are sometimes used in children with TD. Although they are usually effective in managing ADHD symptoms in this group, use of stimulants may result in an increase in tic symptoms. Symptoms of OCD can also be treated with medications such as the SSRIs.

> Isaiah is an 8-year-old boy in the third grade. He first developed tics when he was 5 years old. At first, his tics included eye blinking, head jerks, facial grimaces, and squinting. Now, he also has several vocal tics including throat clearing and snorting. Like many children with TD, Isaiah also has ADHD and is in constant trouble at school. He gets sent out of class at least once a week and has been suspended five times in the last 6 months. Infractions include disruptive classroom behavior such as making animal sounds in class and disrespectful behavior such as making pelvic thrusting movements toward the teacher. His teacher reports that Isaiah is constantly out of his seat sharpening his pencil or straightening books in the classroom.

Isaiah's problem behaviors are likely part of his disorder. The animal sounds and pelvic thrusts are actually common tics displayed by children his age. It sounds as though Isaiah is also developing symptoms of OCD. He may be unable to stop himself from leaving his seat to engage in compulsions such as pencil sharpening or straightening. It is very important that Isaiah's parents, teachers, and classmates understand that people with TD are often unable to control their tics, even when they are highly motivated to do so. Punishing him by removing him from class or suspending him will not change his behavior and may actually be making his symptoms worse by adding stress. Children with TD tend to have good periods and bad periods, so it may look as though Isaiah has more control over his tics than he actually does. It may help to give Isaiah freedom to leave the room regularly to express tics. A child like Isaiah who has TD along with symptoms of OCD and ADHD will likely require a combination of medications. Further, because TD follows a waxing and waning course, medications may have to be adjusted more frequently than with other disorders.

DEVELOPMENTAL DISABILITIES

Mental Retardation

Children with mental retardation have deficits in intellectual ability and adaptive behaviors. By definition, a child diagnosed with mental retardation must have an IQ below 70 and must have deficits in adaptive functioning in two of the following areas: communication, self-care, home living, social or interpersonal skills, use of community resources, self-direction, functional academic skills, work, leisure, health, and safety. In addition, these problems must begin before the child is 18 years old. People with mental retardation fall into one of four categories: mild (IQ between 50–55 and approximately 70), moderate (IQ between 35–40 and 50–55), severe (IQ between 20–25 and 35–40), and profound (IQ below 20–25).

> Eve is a nonverbal 13-year-old girl with moderate mental retardation. Her behavior at school has become increasingly difficult to manage. She is constantly on the go and has a difficult time sitting in her chair for any length of time. She has been having multiple aggressive outbursts every day and has severely scratched the arms of several teacher's assistants. Her teacher is working with her on a picture exchange system to increase her communication skills, but her aggressive outbursts are limiting the amount of time that can be devoted to educational programming.

Eve needs a functional behavioral assessment to identify the cause of her aggressive outbursts. Eve's teacher should then focus on teaching her an alternative response to scratching in order to meet her needs. It sounds as though her teacher is off to a good start with the picture exchange system. At the same time it may also help to prescribe some medication to decrease hyperactivity and to reduce aggression. An antihypertensive medication such as guanfacine or clonidine might be considered. The addition of medication may allow Eve to benefit more fully from the educational plan her teacher has written so that her communication and coping skills can be improved.

Autism Spectrum Disorders

Autism disorders are also called the pervasive developmental disorders. They include autism, Asperger syndrome, and pervasive developmental disorder not otherwise specified. Autism disorders are characterized by deficits in social interaction skills. Children with autism have three primary characteristics: impairments in social interaction, impairments in communication, and stereotyped behaviors or interests. Social impairments may include a failure to make friends, to show interest in the activities of others, or to seek social companionship. Children with autism often communicate poorly because they fail to use eye contact and facial expressions. They have difficulty understanding social rules and expectations. In the area of communications, some children with autism may fail to develop functional language. Others may use language but may have difficulty with conversational skills and the social use of language. Finally, some children may use language in atypical ways like echoing words or phrases they have heard in the past or using pronouns incorrectly. Stereotyped behaviors range from unusual motor movements (e.g., hand flapping) to perseverative behaviors (e.g., looking at things from odd angles) to obsessive interests (e.g., vacuums, bottle caps, sea creatures). Over 75% of children with autism have cognitive impairments. Others do not have cognitive impairments, and some are even considered to be gifted. Therefore, a diagnosis of autism does not mean that the child also has mental retardation.

Children with Asperger syndrome have social deficits similar to those of children with autism. They may fail to understand social interactions and may have a difficult time making and maintaining friends. They also display similar stereotyped behaviors including obsessive interests, rigid adherence to routine, and unusual motor movements. However, children with Asperger syndrome do not have delays in communication or self-help skills. By definition their cognitive abilities do not fall in the impaired range.

Pervasive developmental disorder not otherwise specified (PDDNOS) is diagnosed when a child has some of the features of Asperger syndrome and autism but does not meet strict diagnostic criteria for these disorders.

J. J. is a 12-year-old boy with Asperger syndrome who is in a mainstream seventh-grade program. Although J. J. has always suffered from obsessive interests, his current obsession with earthquakes is significantly interfering with his academic performance. He often insists on moving his desk away from windows and into the classroom doorway in case there is an earthquake. He talks so much about earthquakes that he is not completing his work and everyone in the school is tired of hearing earthquake facts and statistics. He has recently taken to wearing a helmet to school to avoid being hurt in an earthquake, which has made him the target of significant peer teasing. Some students in the school have also discovered that they can upset J. J. by quietly shaking their desks with their knees. Although he is a good student, his teachers feel he may have to move to a self-contained class if these problems continue.

Obsessive interests are common among children with Asperger syndrome. In this case, J. J.'s interests are interfering with his academic and social functioning. In addition, he seems to be living with high levels of anxiety. A trial of a medication used for obsessive–compulsive disorder, such as an SSRI antidepressant, may be helpful.

Children with developmental disabilities are more likely to have behavioral and mood problems than other children. Problems can include aggression, self-injurious behavior, tantrums, and stereotyped behavior. Disruptive behavior may be caused by medical or environmental factors or a combination of the two. In many cases, behavioral problems result when children are unable to communicate their needs to others. Many professionals dismiss emotional and behavioral problems as being part of the child's developmental disability. However, psychiatric problems can limit the child's adaptive functioning as much as the developmental disability itself.

There are no medications that treat the core features of autism disorders or mental retardation. However, medications are frequently used to manage symptoms that interfere with the child's functioning and ability to profit from education. Once a problem has been identified, the same principles that apply to treatment of children without mental retardation are used. However, modifications are often made to match the child's developmental level and communicative ability. Table 4.7 provides an overview of the types of medications used to manage symptoms sometimes seen in children with developmental disabilities.

The success of behavioral treatment programs for individuals with mental retardation and autism spectrum disorders has caused some people to question the use of medications with this population. There has been some concern that medications are used as a first treatment option before other less intrusive methods have been attempted. The best treatment plans often involve a combination of medical, habilitative, and educational interventions.

As with other disorders, the medications used for children are often ones that have been tested primarily with adults. Parents, teachers, and physicians must be especially vigilant in the assessment and monitoring of adverse effects because these children often lack the communication skills needed to alert adults to problems. Extrapyramidal symptoms, tardive dyskinesia, and akathisia can signal serious problems and must be addressed quickly.

Mood problems like depression may occur frequently in children with developmental disabilities but may be difficult to recognize due to communication impairments. The frustrations of trying to get by in the world can lead to sadness and hopelessness. There is some evidence that SSRIs are effective in treating mood problems and impulse control in children and adolescents with developmental disabilities. Similarly, the atypical antidepressants and the atypical antianxiety medications may be effective in treating mood problems, anxiety, and irritability. For children and adolescents with mood swings or cyclic

TABLE 4.7. Medications for Children with Developmental Disabilities, Including Autism Spectrum Disorders and Mental Retardation

Symptom	Medication treatment options
Hyperactivity, impulsivity, inattention	Stimulants, antihypertensives
Obsessive–compulsive behaviors	SSRIs, antidepressants
Aggression	Antihypertensives, beta blockers, benzodiazepines, antipsychotics
Self-injury	Antihypertensives, beta blockers, benzodiazepines, antipsychotics, naltrexone
Depression	SSRI antidepressants, tricyclic antidepressants
Anxiety	SSRI antidepressants
Stereotyped or repetitive behaviors	SSRI antidepressants
Mood swings	Lithium, antiepileptics

mood disorders such as bipolar disorder, lithium and antiepileptic medications may be helpful in treating symptoms like mood cycling, irritability, and aggression.

ADHD is a common problem for children and adolescents with developmental disabilities. Symptoms such as impulsivity, inattention, and hyperactivity can significantly affect the child's ability to benefit from educational programming. ADHD medications can exert similar effects on children with and without developmental disabilities. However, there is some evidence that children with developmental disabilities may have more adverse effects and that lower-functioning children may benefit less from medication than higher-functioning children.

Disruptive behaviors like aggression and self-injury are among the most troubling problems seen in children and adolescents with developmental disabilities. Successful treatment of disruptive behavior often determine whether the child should be cared for at home or can attend a neighborhood school. Behavioral treatments are considered to be the best first intervention in treating disruptive behaviors in children with developmental disabilities. The first part of a behavioral treatment is conducting a functional behavior assessment. The treatment designed is based on the assessment. Treatment plans usually involve teaching new adaptive skills to replace disruptive behaviors.

When behavioral treatment plans are ineffective or when the behavior is physically damaging (e.g., head banging), medications are often prescribed. However, medication should not be prescribed in the absence of a companion behavior management program. Medications, however, are very effective in treating severe disruptive behavior in children with developmental disabilities. Atypical antipsychotics such as risperidone and olanzapine have been successfully used to treat aggression and self-injurious behavior and are usually preferable to older antipsychotics because they pose less risk of long-term side effects. Side effects of these medications can include weight gain and sedation. Tardive dyskinesia and neuroleptic malignant syndrome are unlikely but possible. In some cases of significant self-injurious behaviors, opiate blockers such as naltrexone can be helpful. In addition, there is some evidence that naltrexone may reduce hyperactivity and aggression and improve communication and prosocial behavior. Antiepileptic medications can be helpful in stabilizing mood and preventing rage episodes. Side effects can include drowsiness, tearfulness, and possibly increased aggression.

Perseverative, obsessive–compulsive, and stereotyped behaviors are often treated with SSRIs. Antihypertensive medications have also been useful in reducing stereotyped motor movements, self-stimulatory behavior, and hyperactivity. However, sedation and fatigue can result.

PSYCHOTIC DISORDERS

Psychotic symptoms include hallucinations (seeing things that are not there) and delusions (false beliefs). Hallucinations can be auditory (e.g., hearing voices), visual (e.g., seeing ghosts or shadows), tactile (e.g., feeling crawling sensations on the skin), or olfactory (e.g., smelling rancid garbage). Examples of delusions include believing that someone is following the family, believing that there is a child trapped in the walls of the house, or believing that the child's parents have been replaced by robots. Children experiencing psychotic symptoms may not always report these symptoms to parents and teachers. Some children with psychosis may have disorganized behavior and may have intense outbursts. They may use disorganized speech that doesn't make sense or language that seems to go off on tangents and is difficult to follow. Other children may become withdrawn and show little emotion (i.e., flat affect). These children may avoid eye contact and may be unresponsive. Unlike the symptoms seen in autism spectrum disorders, which are usually apparent by 18 months of age and improve over time, the symptoms seen in psychotic disorders tend to begin later in childhood or adolescence and tend to become worse over time.

Psychotic symptoms can occur during the course of a medical condition or in reaction to substance use. When symptoms occur for 6 months or more and no other cause can be identified, schizophrenia may be present. Psychotic disorders are typically not diagnosed in children younger than 7. Symptoms usually begin in the late teens, although signs of psychiatric problems may be identifiable at an earlier age. It is very rare for a child under the age of 10 to be diagnosed with a psychotic disorder. Childhood onset of psychotic symptoms tends to predict a more severe form of the disorder and a worse prognosis than later onset.

Psychotherapy is generally not an effective treatment for psychosis. Family therapy is often used to decrease stress in the home, which can help control the symptoms. Table 4.8 provides an overview of the medications used to treat psychotic disorders in children. Atypical antipsychotics are usually the first medications prescribed for a child with psychosis. These include risperidone, olanzapine, and quetiapine. These medications may have

TABLE 4.8. Medications for the Management of Psychotic Disorders in Children

Generic (trade) name	Class	Side effects
Haloperidol (Haldol)	Antipsychotic	Can cause sedation, weight gain, cognitive blunting, decreased seizure threshold; must monitor for movement disorders.
Loxapine (Loxitane)	Antipsychotic	Can cause sedation, weight gain, cognitive blunting, decreased seizure threshold; must monitor for movement disorders.
Thioridazine (Mellaril)	Antipsychotic	Can cause sedation, weight gain, cognitive blunting, decreased seizure threshold; must monitor for movement disorders.
Thiothixene (Navane)	Antipsychotic	Can cause sedation, weight gain, cognitive blunting, decreased seizure threshold; must monitor for movement disorders.
Clozapine (Clozaril)	Atypical antipsychotic	Can cause sedation, weight gain, cognitive blunting, decreased seizure threshold; must monitor for movement disorders; can result in fatal drops in bone marrow and white blood cell count.
Olanzapine (Zyprexa)	Atypical antipsychotic	Can cause sedation, weight gain, cognitive blunting, decreased seizure threshold; must monitor for movement disorders.
Risperidone (Risperdal)	Atypical antipsychotic	Can cause sedation, weight gain, cognitive blunting, decreased seizure threshold; must monitor for movement disorders.
Quetiapine (Seroquel)	Atypical antipsychotic	Can cause sedation, weight gain, cognitive blunting, decreased seizure threshold; must monitor for movement disorders.

fewer side effects (and less dangerous side effects) than the traditional antipsychotics. They may also treat negative symptoms of schizophrenia, such as flat facial expressions, lack of speech, and poor engagement in activities. These medications can result in sedation, anticholinergic effects (constipation, blurred vision, dry eyes, dry mouth), or extrapyramidal side effects (tremors, spasms, balance problems). These side effects are usually much milder than those encountered with traditional antipsychotics.

The traditional antipsychotics (e.g., haloperidol) are often used when the newer atypical medications are not effective. Children taking these medications must be monitored carefully because there is a risk of developing extrapyramidal symptoms, such as involuntary movements, tremors, muscle spasms, and balance problems.

In addition to prescribing an antipsychotic medication to treat psychotic symptoms in children, the physician may add a second or third medication to help treat symptoms of mood instability, aggression, or anxiety.

Marcus is a 17-year-old male in his senior year of high school. He has always been a quiet, shy student who has received B's and C's in his classes. However, over the past few months, Marcus has become increasingly withdrawn and has been observed sitting by himself at lunch. He has been coming to school looking disheveled and he seems to be wearing the same T-shirt to school every day. Although he has never been a stellar student, his performance has decreased dramatically. He has been turning in homework that is half finished with answers that do not make sense. His English teacher finally decided to call his parents when he turned in a 22-page poem that was written in tiny handwriting and seemed to be about the president and the seven deadly sins.

Marcus's behavior may be consistent with the early stages of schizophrenia (the prodromal phase). During this phase, the adolescent may become socially isolated and start to show unusual behaviors. His performance in school may decline, and he may start to neglect self-care. Marcus's poem may reflect the beginning of what is called the active phase of a psychotic disorder, where the individual starts to hear voices, see things that are not there, or form irrational or bizarre beliefs. Marcus's teacher did the right thing by calling his mother. His mother should take him to his primary care physician immediately for evaluation. With proper diagnosis and treatment, Marcus's symptoms will likely improve.

EATING AND ELIMINATION DISORDERS

Eating Disorders

The two major types of eating disorders are anorexia nervosa and bulimia nervosa. People with anorexia are afraid of gaining weight. They maintain a weight that is below normal for their height. While teenagers and adults with anorexia usually lose a lot of weight, some children with anorexia will fail to gain weight at the expected rate. Most people with anorexia continue to believe they are overweight even when they are very thin. Girls with anorexia usually stop having their menstrual periods or fail to have periods in the first place. People with anorexia may limit their food intake, exercise excessively, or vomit after eating in order to maintain a low body weight.

Individuals with bulimia nervosa engage in disordered episodes of binge eating. A binge involves eating a very large amount of food in a short period of time (less than 2 hours). Individuals with bulimia then attempt to prevent weight gain from the binge episode by vomiting, using laxatives, fasting, or exercising excessively. Children and adolescents with bulimia can be more difficult to identify than those with anorexia because they do not necessarily maintain an extremely low body weight.

Both anorexia and bulimia are very serious and dangerous disorders that need to be addressed quickly. In addition to the risk of death, these eating disorders are associated with long-term and irreversible damage to the body. Family and individual psychotherapy are typically used to treat eating disorders. Antidepressant medications can also be effective as an adjunct to psychological treatment. SSRIs are often prescribed for individuals with eating disorders. When children and adolescents with eating disorders have co-occurring problems like depression, anxiety, or excessive mood instability, these problems may also be treated with medications.

> Amanda is a 13-year-old girl who is in the eighth grade. She has always been an excellent student who usually receives top grades and excels in sports. Her gym teacher has noticed that she is much quieter and less social this year than she was in the seventh grade. Although she usually wears baggy clothes and changes in a bathroom stall when she has gym class, her teacher is becoming increasingly aware that Amanda's weight is abnormally low. When she asks Amanda's friends, they report that she usually goes to club meetings or extra band practices during lunchtime, so they are not sure whether she is eating.

It is not unusual for people with anorexia to hide weight loss by wearing baggy clothes and avoiding changing in public places. Similarly, Amanda may be arranging her schedule so that she does not have to face her friends during lunchtime. It is very important that Amanda's gym teacher share her concerns with Amanda's parents. Depending on her current weight and the seriousness of her physical condition, Amanda may need immediate medical attention, including possible stabilization in a hospital. If she is diagnosed with anorexia nervosa, she will likely require intensive treatment, including family therapy and individual therapy. The school can help by giving Amanda ways to make up work she misses during her treatment that are attainable and fair. If she misses a significant amount of school, extra tutoring or home instruction may be needed. It also sounds as though Amanda may be suffering from depression. She might benefit from treatment with a medication that treats these symptoms.

Elimination Disorders

Most young children have occasional daytime or nighttime toileting accidents. However, children who continue to have regular urine accidents after the age of 5 may have enuresis. Enuresis is typically diagnosed when the child has at least two accidents per week for 3 or more months.

Enuresis can occur during sleep (nocturnal enuresis) or during the day (diurnal enuresis). Daytime accidents are less common and may be a sign of a physical problem. Children with daytime accidents may have urinary tract infections that require antibiotics. They may also benefit from antispasmodic medications to reduce bladder contractions.

Bedwetting (nocturnal enuresis) is a more common problem and affects about 1 in 10 school-age children. Although no physical cause for the problem can be identified in most cases, scientists believe bedwetting may be related to antidiuretic hormones, poor muscle control, delays in nervous system development, or emotional problems. There is evidence of a strong genetic component to bedwetting.

Enuresis can be treated behaviorally or medically. The TCA imipramine was once frequently used to treat bedwetting. However, because of the risk of serious cardiac problems related to this medication, it is no longer commonly used. Desmopressin (DDAVP) is a synthetic hormone that can be taken as either a nasal spray or a tablet and is effective in treating enuresis. Unfortunately, many children return to bedwetting once they discontinue DDAVP.

Behavioral treatments for bedwetting usually include a urine alarm system that trains the child to wake up before full urination by sounding an alarm when the first few drops appear (this treatment works through avoidance conditioning). More than 75% of children with bedwetting can be successfully treated using a urine alarm. The urine alarm system is often combined with other behavioral treatments, such as cleanliness training (having the child change underwear and sheets following an accident) and retention control (teaching the child to postpone urination to build urinary muscles). To prevent relapse once the urine alarm system is discontinued, physicians recommend that the child practice urinating at night by drinking liquids shortly before bedtime (overlearning).

Some children have accidents involving bowel movements. When this occurs at least once per month for 3 months past the age of 4, this disorder is called encopresis. In many cases, encopresis is related to constipation. In these cases, the child's colon becomes impacted and feces leak around the impaction and into the child's underpants. When severe constipation has persisted for a long time, the child's colon may lose muscle tone, making it even more difficult for the child to prevent accidents. These accidents are not under the child's control and it is important to remember the child is not willfully soiling pants or not cleaning after toileting. When constipation is involved, it is important to treat this aspect of the problem first through the use of laxatives, enemas, dietary changes, and stool softeners. Medications alone are usually not sufficient to treat encopresis. A behavioral program is recommended to reward the child for sitting on the toilet, defecating in the toilet, and having clean underpants. Skills training to teach body cues associated with defecation and to teach discrimination of the correct place to defecate is also helpful. Punishment or overcorrection procedures may also be helpful.

April is a 9-year-old girl with PDDNOS who is in a mainstream third-grade class. Her teacher has noticed that someone in the class has been smearing feces on the walls of the bathroom stall in the girls' restroom. After watching the class and checking the bathroom frequently, she is fairly sure that April is the child.

April's teacher needs to share this information with her parents and suggest that they take her to her pediatrician. Feces-smearing can occur when a child is unable to control her bowels due to severe constipation. This can result in stains in the child's underwear as well as leakage of actual fecal matter. April may be trying to clean off her underpants (and then her hands) during trips to the bathroom. Because she has PDDNOS, she may have difficulty communicating her symptoms to her parents and teacher. If April does have encopresis, she will likely require medical treatment for constipation. Some children who have been chronically constipated may be fearful of having bowel movements because they have been painful in the past. April's teacher may be asked to send her to the bathroom to sit on the toilet for specific periods during the day. Parents may also be asked to include high-fiber foods for April's lunch and to reward her for drinking lots of water.

SUMMARY

There are numerous psychotropic medications that are frequently used for many psychiatric disorders, including problems associated with attention, disruptive behavior disorders, anxiety disorders, mood disorders, tic disorders, developmental disabilities, psychotic disorders, and disorders of eating and elimination. Frequently, these disorders may occur together as do anxiety and mood disorders. Teachers and parents can be valuable informants of specific symptoms that may facilitate the diagnosis of one or more of these disorders. There are a number of treatments available that typically include either psychosocial treatments used alone or a combination of medication and psychosocial treatments.

REFERENCES

American Psychiatric Association. (2000). *Diagnostic and statistical manual of mental disorders* (4th ed., text rev.). Washington, DC: Author.

Reiff, M. I., & Tippin, S. (2004). *ADHD: A complete authoritative guide.* Elk Grove Village, IL: American Academy of Pediatrics.

5

Medication Effectiveness
and Side Effects

Along with monitoring for adverse side effects, the most important aspect of working with children who are taking psychotropic medications is determining whether or not the medications are effective. Best practice methods that measure medication effectiveness are the focus of this chapter. Evaluation forms that assist in determining whether or not the medications are effective are provided in Appendices 11–15.

A wide range of childhood disorders and problems can be treated effectively with medication. However, and unfortunately, even the best medications sometimes are not effective. In other cases, medication side effects may be difficult to tolerate. For example, Joanie is a 7-year-old girl with mild ADHD. She was prescribed a stimulant to help her focus better in school. Within 2 months of starting the medication, Joanie developed a very distracting throat-clearing tic. In this case, the side effect of the medication was more problematic than the original problem, and Joanie's physician decided to try a different treatment approach.

Predicting how a particular child will respond to a particular medication is very difficult. When children are initially prescribed psychiatric medication, the first few days, weeks, or months are considered a trial period. This means that the child will try the medication for a period of time while the physician and family (including the child) determine whether the medication is a good choice or whether a different approach should be investigated.

School personnel can be important partners during a child's medication trial. They are in a good position to provide other treatment team members information about the child's academic performance, behavior, and social interactions. This is especially important when medications have been prescribed specifically to treat school problems. Clearly, teachers and others who are aware the child has begun taking medications can provide helpful information. Paradoxically, this is also true when school personnel are not told of medication initiation or changes. This allows them an unbiased perspective on the effects of the medication versus expectations that might color their observational opinions. This non-informed status is best sustained only temporarily, however. In many situations, school personnel are often told little about medications the child is taking and physicians are told little about the child's behavior at school. Having these separate worlds of information can lead to ineffective or even harmful treatments.

A frequent question is why school personnel are asked to monitor psychiatric medication but not medications for flu, asthma, or other medical problems. The reason is that the effects of psychiatric medications are not usually as clear as the effects of other types of medications. If you have a rash, you might be given an antihistamine. If the rash disappears, you know that the antihistamine worked. Psychiatric treatment is more difficult to evaluate because the problems are more complex. Also, many symptoms appear along a continuum from tolerable to necessitating rapid intervention. Many symptoms treated with psychiatric medications are not as obvious as a rash. Problems might be somewhat difficult to determine. How do you know if a child is overly anxious or just temporarily scared? When problems are hard to define, it is difficult to decide whether they have gotten worse or better. In addition, unlike a medication that makes a rash disappear, many psychiatric medications don't eliminate problems completely. Instead, they may make the problem less noticeable or troublesome. It is harder to tell if a problem has gotten better than if it has resolved completely.

Taking medications can involve risks of side effects and always involves money and other resources. If the medication is effective, these risks and costs are often acceptable. If the medication does not improve the symptoms, the risks and costs are not acceptable. Treatment monitoring can help physicians decide to continue a medication or try other approaches.

When scientists study the effects of medications, they often compare the response of children taking the medication to the response of children taking an inactive compound called a placebo. A placebo is a pill that does not contain any medication but looks like a pill that does. It generally contains inert compounds (like sugar, for instance) that have no effect on the body. When evaluating the efficacy of medications, it is important to consider placebo effects. This allows the scientists to evaluate how much of the medication's effectiveness is due to its chemical actions and how much is due to other factors associated with taking it. The placebo effect can be very powerful. In some cases, although there is no medicinal value in a placebo pill, as much as 50% of the improvement seen in some patients is attributed to the placebo effect. Some side effects are also the result of the placebo effect, just as if the person were taking medication.

Placebo effects may be due to a person's belief that a treatment will work. In some cases, strong beliefs may affect a person's brain chemistry and may cause changes in the way the person feels and behaves. In other cases, people in the child's environment may treat the child differently because they know that the child is taking a medication, which, in turn, can result in changes in the child's behavior. Physicians, parents, or teachers may look for positive changes when they know that a child is taking medication and may notice behaviors that they might not have noticed before the child started taking medication. This occurs in day-to-day life just as it does in scientific trials. The placebo effect is one reason that monitoring treatment effectiveness using the methods described in this chapter is so important.

When a child begins a new psychiatric medication, effective monitoring may be neglected. Often, the physician will simply ask the parent whether the child seems better. The parent might ask the teacher and they might agree that the child seems to be doing better. There are two problems with this undefined approach. First, because of the placebo effect, people might think the child is doing better when no change has occurred. Second, the physician might think the child is receiving the best medication or the best dose of medication for the problem when in fact a different medication or dose might work better. In the following sections, we outline a systematic approach for monitoring treatment effects. Five steps used in monitoring a treatment are outlined: identifying the treatment goals, identifying problem behaviors, tracking behaviors, graphing results, and monitoring side effects. Reproducible forms are included to help the observer with each step of the process.

IDENTIFYING TREATMENT GOALS

To some people, this step might seem obvious. The goal of treatment is to make the child better. However, there are many ways to define "better." For some children, the treatment goal might be to improve academic performance. For others, the goal might be to decrease aggressive behavior. Making the goals clear allows a more accurate assessment of whether a medication is effective. It is also important that families, physicians, and school personnel be open and honest with each other about what they expect the medication will do for the child. If a child is being aggressive at school, it is important that parents and physicians know that this is the primary concern. The child may also be inattentive, but giving a child the medication for inattention is unlikely to affect the child biting other children.

Gabriel, a 10-year-old boy with autism, is an excellent example of the need to identify treatment goals. Gabriel's parents brought him to a child psychiatrist because they were receiving frequent reports from his school about his aggressive behavior. Rather than putting him on medication for aggression, Gabriel's psychiatrist decided to talk to his teacher about the problem. The teacher let the psychiatrist know that Gabriel was making frequent verbal threats to other children in the class, but he had never actually attacked anyone. Although clearly a concern, his aggressive behavior was more disruptive than dangerous. The teacher also reported that Gabriel seemed very anxious at school in unfamiliar situations. This information helped Gabriel's psychiatrist choose a medication that reduced anxiety and in turn reduced Gabriel's verbal threats.

If school personnel are asked to monitor changes in a child's behavior, ask the parent what problems the medication is supposed to reduce. Common problems include attention, hyperactivity, tics, impulsivity, aggression, angry outbursts, and self-injurious behavior.

Angela is a 4-year-old girl with developmental delays. She is very active and her teacher has a difficult time getting her to stay in her chair. She often leaves the designated area during activities and has to be monitored closely. She also can be aggressive with other children and adults. She bites other children at least once per week. Her physician has decided to give Angela a trial of a stimulant medication and asks her teacher, Mr. Shields, to provide feedback about her behavior. Because Mr. Shields is concerned about both biting and hyperactivity, he needs to clarify the treatment goal. After talking with Angela's parents, he learns the medication has been prescribed to decrease hyperactivity. Therefore, the behavior Mr. Shields needs to monitor is activity level.

SELECTING BEHAVIORS TO MONITOR

Once the treatment goal has been identified, specific problem behaviors should be identified. Monitoring these behaviors will help evaluate movement toward the treatment goals, so the behaviors should reflect the treatment goals. If the goal is to improve academic performance, the behaviors monitored might include scores on spelling tests or grades on written assignments.

Other behaviors are more difficult to monitor. Everyone knows what being silly is. However, it is hard to keep track of how silly children are, how often they are silly, and whether a medication is working to make them less silly. This is because different people have different ideas of what silly is. Silly is sometimes a good thing and sometimes a bad thing, so it can be hard to pinpoint when being silly is a problem. Other behaviors that are difficult to track include being nice, feeling confident, and acting happy. Deciding how to define such ways of being or acting is important in measuring them. Taking time to get an operational definition of a behavior is worth the effort.

Table 5.1 provides some examples of behaviors you might choose to monitor. They are divided into four categories: academic behaviors, problem behaviors, positive behaviors, and peer interactions. Of course, there are countless behaviors that can be monitored, so this table is merely a starting point. The type of behavior you choose to measure will depend on the goal of treatment and on what is possible and practical for a teacher to monitor.

To monitor medication effectiveness, choose behaviors that are easy to define and measure and can be defined very precisely. Once a definition has been written, even a substitute teacher should be able to look at the definition and evaluate the child's behavior without further instruction. Anyone who has ever been around children knows what a temper tantrum is. However, "temper tantrum" can be surprisingly difficult to define. A behavior that one person might define as a temper tantrum might only be loud crying to another person. In addition, the same behavior might be tolerable on easy days but might be called a temper tantrum when the day has been difficult and the adult in the room is stressed. How the behavior is defined is less important than its being defined so that it is easy to evaluate and measure and reflects the goal of treatment. Some examples of good definitions for temper tantrums include:

TABLE 5.1. Behaviors to Monitor

Area	Behavior examples
Academic performance	Number of problems completed in a 5-minute period
	Number of worksheets completed in a half-hour period
	Scores on weekly spelling or arithmetic tests
	Amount of time it takes to complete one reading assignment and answer questions
	Number of loose papers in desk and backpack
Problem behaviors	How often a tic occurs
	How often the child hits, kicks, or bites others
	Number of time-outs (the behaviors for which a child is placed in time-out must be well defined)
	Number of times a child is out of seat without permission
	Number or length of tantrums
	Length of time spent crying each day (or number of episodes)
Positive behaviors	How often the child raises a hand to respond to a question
	How many times per day a child laughs
	Number of times per week the child turns in homework
	Length of time the child spends on-task during an activity
Peer interactions	Number of minutes spent playing with others during recess
	Number of disagreements or fights with peers

- Child cries for more than 30 seconds.
- Child falls on the ground and protests for any amount of time.
- Child screams for 1 minute or more.
- Child cries for at least 5 minutes and screams at least once.

Again, any definition for temper tantrum is acceptable (including ones that are not on this list) as long as it is easy to recognize, precise, and easy to communicate.

Some people worry that keeping track of behaviors is too much work in the midst of other duties. However, tracking behaviors might be easier than you think. Below is a list of ways to monitor behaviors. Be creative in generating methods to gather information that are useful but interfere only marginally with your other work.

1. Take photographs. This works especially well for evidence of self-injurious behaviors, such as calluses and bruises left from hand mouthing or skin picking. Take a picture of the worst area on the child's body every day or every week. Then compare the pictures across time to see if the injuries are decreasing. Self-injurious and other-injurious behaviors are the most important ones to control. First, however, determine school policy about taking photographs, get permission from parents and assent from the child (if possible), and use signed releases if appropriate. These could be included as part of the overall treatment plan.

2. Measure performance in a task that is done once per day or per week. This allows you to keep careful track of a behavior without having to pay attention all day. Rather than making a half-hearted attempt to track the child's behavior all day, do a good job of moni-

toring the behavior for a short time (usually between 5 and 60 minutes) once per day or week. The behavior observation forms in Appendices 11–13 will simplify this effort.

    a. How many times does Bethany leave her chair during silent reading each day?
    b. How many problems can John finish during a 5-minute speed-arithmetic task?

3. Keep a daily count of the identified behaviors. Rather than trying to keep track of lots of behaviors, just chose one or two to track over several weeks.

    a. How many times per day does Jill raise her hand?
    b. How many times per week does Roger bite other students?
    c. How many times per day does James cry?
    d. How many recesses does Rachel miss each week for any reason?

4. For severely inattentive and disorganized children, count the number of loose papers inside the child's desk, on the floor around the desk, or in the backpack on a daily or weekly basis.
5. Track grades on weekly exams.
6. Keep a record of homework turned in and completed.

    a. Does the child turn in daily assignment without reminders?
    b. Was the homework assignment completed correctly?

7. Complete a simple rating scale at the end of each day (e.g., worked hard, followed directions, kept hands and feet to self). If there is an assistant who works with the child, consider not informing the assistant about the child's medication changes but have the assistant complete the daily checklist. This will allow for unbiased monitoring of behavior.

Mei is a 6-year-old girl with social phobia and separation anxiety disorder. Since starting the first grade, she barely talks in class unless she is one-on-one with a teacher or another student. Her physician has decided to prescribe an anxiety medication and has asked her teacher, Ms. Phillips, to provide feedback about whether the medication is helping. Ms. Phillips has 25 first graders in her class, so she needs to choose a behavior that is easy to monitor. She decides to monitor verbal behavior during circle time, which lasts for 20 minutes each morning. During this period, the children are expected to greet each other. They are also called on to answer questions and to share stories. She decides to keep track of the number of words Mei says during circle time each day. (This would work best for low verbalizers.) Ms. Phillips knows that Mei will often mouth the words *yes* and *no*, so she determines that in order for a response to count as a word, Mei must say it loud enough for the group to hear. She defines the behavior as "the number of words Mei says during circle time that are audible to the group." At first, Mei only says hello and fails to contribute anything else, even when she is called on (an average of one word per circle time). Over time, however, she begins to respond to direct questions with an audible *yes* or *no* (an average of four words per circle time).

TRACKING BEHAVIORS

Once you have selected an appropriate behavior to track and defined it precisely, you need to find a way to keep track of that behavior. There are many ways to track behaviors. The three most common ways to track behaviors are:

1. *Frequency:* the number of times a behavior occurs in a certain amount of time. Examples include the number of worksheets completed in an hour, the number of times a child cries in a day, and the number of eye tics a child has in a 5-minute period.
2. *Duration:* how long a behavior lasts. Examples include how long a child stays in the chair, how long it took a child to complete a reading task, and how long a child plays appropriately with others.
3. *Percentage correct:* the number of correct responses divided by the number of opportunities. This is the type of information most frequently collected by schools. For example, if a child takes a math test with 100 problems and gets 80 correct, the percentage correct is 80 divided by 100, or 80%.

We have provided three examples of data sheets for tracking behaviors: Behavior Observation Forms 1 through 3 (Appendices 11 through 13). Table 5.2 will help you select the behavior observation form most appropriate for the behavior you would like to monitor. If you have selected percentage correct as the measure, use only Appendix 14 (see the section on graphing results, later in this chapter).

TABLE 5.2. Choosing the Best Behavior Observation Form

Behavior	Behavior Observation Forms 1–3 (Appendices 11–13)
Crying	Event (1) or Duration (2)
Following directions	Event (1)
Head banging	Event (1)
Hitting	Event (1)
In seat	Duration (2)
Number of math problems completed	Event (1)
Number of worksheets completed	Event (1)
Participation in game	Total Duration (3)
Responding to questions	Event (1)
Rocking	Total Duration (3)
Screaming	Event (1) or Total Duration (3)
Obsessive talking about a topic	Event (1) or Total Duration (3)
Talking without raising hand	Event (1)
Throat clearing	Event (1)
Vocal tic	Event (1)
Working on-task	Duration (2)

Behavior Observation Form 1

Behavior Observation Form 1 (Appendix 11) can be used to monitor behaviors like the number of times a child raises a hand, leaves the seat, asks for help, or interrupts. It is not necessary to watch the child all day long to collect this type of information. You can also adjust the length of the observation period depending on the behavior. If it is a behavior that does not happen very often (explosive tantrums), chose a long observation period such as the entire day or the entire afternoon. If it is a behavior that happens often (repetitive eye blinking), choose a short observation period like 5 minutes. Try to use the same length observation period each day and observe at the same times each day. This will allow you to compare your tallies across days. If you decide to monitor hand raising, for example, do it at roughly the same time every day and for about the same length of time each day. That way, if you see an increase or decrease in the behavior, you will know it is likely due to the medication and not to a shorter observation period or changes in the child's behavior at different times of the day.

Many teachers will find that using hash marks for tracking behaviors on the behavior observation form is simple. However, if you must move around while you are observing (such as during an unstructured activity like recess) or if the behavior happens very frequently, it may be easier to keep track of the number of times the behavior occurs by using a wrist or hand counter. Wrist or hand counters are often available at sporting goods stores and have a button that can be depressed each time the behavior is observed. At the end of the observation period, you can simply note the total number of times the behavior occurred on the form. Figure 5.1 is an example of a completed Behavior Observation Form 1.

Ms. Peaks was asked to monitor the behavior of 9-year-old Crystal before and after a change in Crystal's ADHD medication. The goal of treatment was to decrease hyperactivity. Ms. Peaks decided to track two of Crystal's behaviors: getting out of her seat without permission and talking without raising her hand. Because these were behaviors that happened often, Ms. Peaks decided to observe Crystal for 45 minutes each morning during math period. During the first week of observation, Crystal took her old medication. On average, she talked without raising her hand six times in each observation period and got out of her seat twice in each observation period. During the second week of observation, Crystal started her new medication. On average, she talked without raising her hand twice in each observation period and got out of her seat without permission twice. These results are graphed in Figures 5.2 and 5.3.

Behavior Observation Form 2

Behavior Observation Form 2 (Appendix 12) can be used to keep track of behaviors that are difficult to count, like rocking. The form is used to track the length of a behavior. It can be used to keep track of the length of tantrums or the amount of time a child sits in a chair without getting up. A stopwatch is the easiest way to track the tantrum length. When the

Behavior Observation Form 1: Event Recording

Behavior 1: _Talking without raising hand_

Behavior 2: _Getting out of seat without permission_

Date	Observation start time	Observation end time	Behavior 1	Behavior 2
1/15 Monday	9:30	10:14	~~||||~~		||
1/16 Tuesday	9:32	10:13	~~||||~~		
1/17 Wednesday	9:28	10:17	~~||||~~		|||
1/18 Thursday	9:30	10:15	~~||||~~		||
1/19 Friday	10:00	10:28	||||	||
1/22 Monday	9:30	10:17	||		
1/23 Tuesday	9:27	10:15	||||	
1/24 Wednesday	9:31	10:15	||	
1/25 Thursday	9:33	10:15	||||		
1/26 Friday	10:01	10:30	||	

FIGURE 5.1. Example of completed Behavior Observation Form 1.

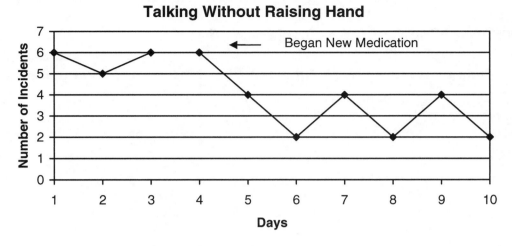

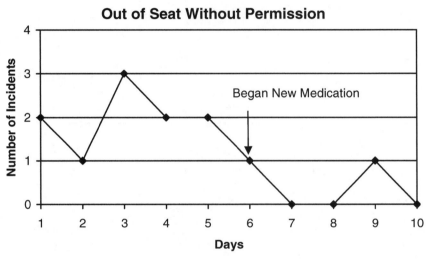

FIGURES 5.2 and 5.3. Examples of data collected using Behavior Observation Form 1.

behavior begins, start the stopwatch. When it ends, stop the stopwatch and write the amount of time on the form. Figure 5.4 is an example of a completed Behavior Observation Form 2.

Jason is an 8-year-old boy who has been having a great deal of difficulty interacting with peers. Mr. Hilton has been asked to keep track of Jason's interactions with others. He decides that he will conduct one observation per recess during which time he will ask another child to go play with Jason. He will then time how long Jason plays with the child before he walks away to do something different. The results, graphed in Figure 5.5, show that Jason is slowly increasing the amount of time he will play following initiation by another child.

Behavior Observation Form 2: Duration Recording

Behavior: *Plays with a peer following an invitation by the peer*

Date	Time behavior started	Time behavior ended	Duration (minutes)
4/3	10:15	10:17	2
4/3	2:11	2:11	0
4/4	10:16	10:19	3
4/4	12:04	12:05	1
4/4	2:10	2:13	3
4/5	10:14	10:17	3
4/5	2:12	2:17	5
4/6	10:10	10:11	4
4/9	10:10	10:17	7
4/9	12:11	12:16	5
4/9	2:05	2:20	15

FIGURE 5.4. Example of completed Behavior Observation Form 2.

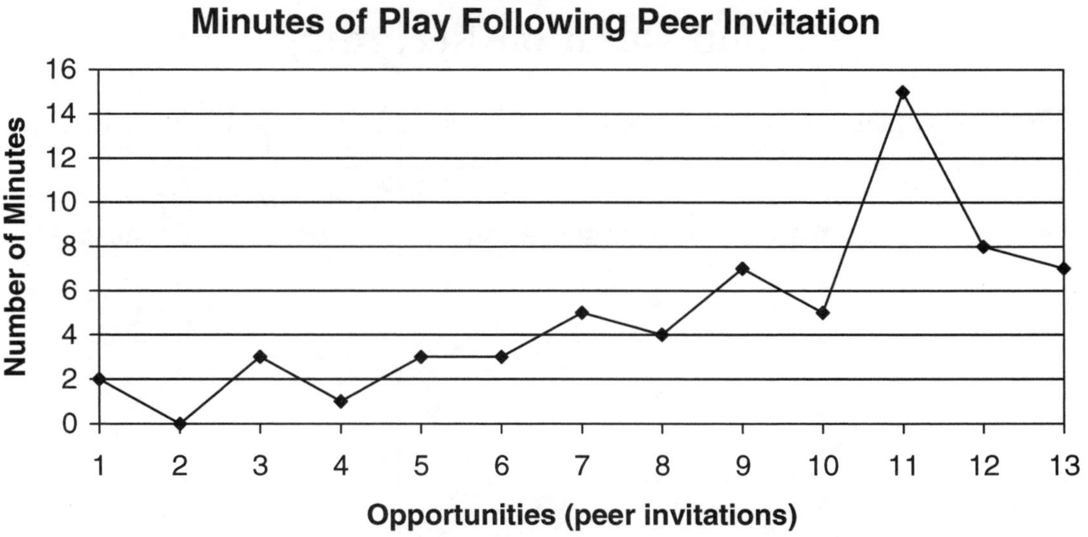

Minutes of Play Following Peer Invitation

FIGURE 5.5. Example of data collected using Behavior Observation Form 2.

Behavior Observation Form 3

Behavior Observation Form 3 (Appendix 13) is used to track the total length of a behavior during a certain period. For example, if you are interested in keeping track of in-seat behavior during a half-hour art activity, start the stopwatch at the beginning of the half hour. Each time the child gets out of the seat, stop the stopwatch. When the child returns to the seat, resume timing. At the end of the half hour, stop the stopwatch. It will show how much time the child has spent seated. Figure 5.6 is an example of a completed Behavior Observation Form 3.

> Chris is a 12-year-old boy with ADHD who is frequently off task during work times. He often does not complete assigned activities because he is talking to other students, fiddling with materials in his backpack, or looking for missing materials. His teacher has been asked to track his attention because he is being considered for ADHD medication. She decides to record on-task behavior during study hall, a 45-minute period that takes place after lunch each day. She defines on-task behavior as sitting in a chair and working on a task (reading or writing). She obtains a stopwatch to record Chris's behavior. At the beginning of study hall, she starts the watch. Each time he talks to a neighbor, gets up to get a drink, stares at the wall, fiddles with materials in his backpack, or does other off-task behaviors, she stops the stopwatch. After 1 week, she finds that Chris is on task for only 11 minutes of each 45-minute study hall period. This is important information she can share with Chris, his parents, and his doctors.

Behavior Observation Form 3:
Total Duration Recording

Behavior: *Stays on task, sitting in seat and reading or writing*

Date	Total time of observation	Total time engaged in target behavior (minutes)
5/4	45	9
5/5	45	11
5/6	45	13
5/7	45	9
5/8	45	12

FIGURE 5.6. Example of Completed Behavior Observation Form 3.

GRAPHING RESULTS

There are many ways to communicate the observation results. A simple line graph is an easy and effective method. A line graph involves a horizontal line that shows time (sessions or days) and a vertical line that shows amount (number, frequency, etc.). Most data collected for medication management purposes can be plotted on the graphs provided in Appendices 14 and 15. Use Line Graph 1 (Appendix 14) to keep track of behaviors that happen 20 or fewer times during an observation period. Use Line Graph 2 (Appendix 15) for behaviors that happen more than 20 times in an observation period. Line Graph 2 can also be used for percentages.

Once the appropriate graph has been selected, give the graph a title so that others will understand what has been graphed. A good title might be: "Number of times [student name] [behavior] during [observation period]" (for example, "Number of times Claire hit her hand on her desk during speech class").

After titling the graph, fill in the data that have been collected. Make a dot on the graph for each day or session you have observed the child. For example, if Claire hit her hand on her desk six times during the first session, make a dot above the 1 (horizontal) and next to the 6 (vertical). Once you have filled in all the data points (up to 19 per graph), connect each dot to the next dot using a straight line. This method will allow you to determine visually whether there has been a change in the child's behavior. You may also wish to draw an arrow to indicate when medication was changed. If you want to show more than 19 days or sessions, use multiple copies of Line Graph 1 or Line Graph 2.

MONITORING ADVERSE EFFECTS

All medications have some potential for creating side effects. Certain side effects are associated with certain medications or classes of medications. Like efficacy, side effects can vary from child to child. One child might experience significant side effects from a certain medication, and another child might be relatively unaffected. There are many different ways to monitor and rate side effects. A child's physician may ask for feedback about side effects. The Side Effects form (Appendix 16) can be used to communicate your observations to parents and physicians.

Remember that children and adolescents may not complain about physical problems and may have difficulty describing physical concerns. Many children, especially those with communication impairments, may require more careful observation when starting a new medication or changing dosages.

SUMMARY

This chapter has described a methodology for monitoring medications in school-age children. The process involves five sequential steps:

1. Identify treatment goals.
2. Choose behaviors to monitor.
3. Monitor behaviors.
4. Graph results.
5. Monitor adverse effects.

This type of monitoring system can play a vital role in ensuring that children are receiving the best medication and the best dosage to improve learning, behavior, and quality of life. Classroom observations provide excellent opportunities for controlled collection of information on noncompliance, excess motor movement, social interaction, on-task behaviors, and many other types of behavior. Observations during unstructured activities like recess can also provide data on appropriate play activities, unstructured social interactions, and play skills. Careful monitoring helps evaluate how a medication is affecting a child physically, behaviorally, cognitively, and emotionally. The information gained assists the other members of the child's treatment team in treatment planning and can result in dramatic improvements in the child's capacity to function.

6

Conclusion

Congratulations. Having read this book, you are better equipped to work with children who have psychiatric disorders. You are a more vigilant monitor of these disorders because you know the symptoms and the contexts in which they usually emerge. Children's problems can receive more rapid and probably more accurate interventions because you have worked to learn about these disorders and psychopharmacological practices that target them.

Treatment usually follows a logical path. After someone notices the child is having a problem, or the child reports a problem to others, a physician and often a psychologist assess the symptoms with assistance from the treatment team members, including school personnel. The child's problem is defined and diagnosed, again with input from the other members of the treatment team, including you, parents, and others. Then pertinent treatments are considered. You will be an integral part of successful implementation of the interventions. You are able to assess what improvements occur as a result of treatment and what side effects may be occurring. You are capable now of more sophisticated observations, making your input more accurate. In addition, the forms in the appendices will help you organize the data that you observe and correct. You are able to monitor reactions to medication, and you have information about the legal and ethical matters inherent in managing medication administration at school.

Be sure to read the "Read This First" section at the beginning of this book to review some of the procedures that are important before you implement the suggestions in this book. For example, the primary care provider (usually a physician but sometimes a psychologist) will diagnose the disorder, but that provider should request information from a number of sources (called multiple informants) to ensure the best treatment plan. There is no richer source of data than school for input on how a child performs on developmental tasks outside the family. Remember your importance in this process. Should you encounter the rare physician who is not interested in your information, you might send the physician a copy of your carefully gathered data and perhaps even the title of this book to show you are more informed and skilled than he or she might think. Remind the physician that getting the best treatment for the child is your only goal, and that you believe the data you are sending will improve the treatment decision.

Our overarching goals for this book are to make you aware of your placement and value as members of the treatment team and to give you information that will help increase your abilities as treatment team members. We all strive to relieve the suffering of children and their families. We know your work in the trenches is difficult and intense. We know you are dedicated to helping children learn, grow, and develop. We hope you feel that we have accomplished our goals for this book. Again, congratulations on your newfound knowledge and abilities.

Glossary

Accumulation—the process of building up levels of a medication.

Addiction—a pattern of drug use that is characterized by compulsive and harmful use of a drug and the tendency to relapse when the drug is withdrawn.

Adverse effects—unwanted physiological, behavioral, or cognitive side effects that are associated with medications.

Agents—chemically active substances.

Agoraphobia—a type of panic disorder where the child may refuse to leave the house.

Anorexia nervosa—an eating disorder characterized by refusing food and being unable to gain weight at the expected rate while maintaining a belief in being overweight.

Anticonvulsants (also called antiepileptics)—medications used to treat seizure disorders that also act as mood stabilizers.

Antipsychotic medications—medications used for treating psychotic symptoms like hallucinations and delusions. Also called neuroleptics.

Asperger syndrome—a developmental disorder characterized by a failure to understand social interactions, difficulty making and maintaining friends, and stereotyped behaviors including obsessive interests, rigid adherence to routine, and unusual motor movements, but not characterized by delays in communication or self-help skills or by impaired cognition.

Ataxia—a lack of coordination.

Attention-deficit/hyperactivity disorder (ADHD)—Inattentive-type ADHD involves poor regulation of attention and includes symptoms like failing to pay close attention to assignments, making careless errors, being poorly organized, and being easily distracted. ADHD, hyperactive–impulsive type, involves symptoms of both hyperactivity (i.e., being restless and fidgety) and impulsivity (i.e., interrupting and having difficulty waiting). The third type is ADHD, combined type, and involves symptoms of the other two.

Autism spectrum disorders—developmental disorders also called the pervasive developmental disorders; autism disorders are characterized by deficits in social interaction skills, including impairments in communication and stereotyped behaviors or interests. Autism disorders include autism, Asperger syndrome, and pervasive developmental disorder not otherwise specified (PDDNOS).

Axons—long, slender branches that project off the cell body of a neuron, or soma, and send information from the soma to other neurons.

Baseline level—the intensity or number of symptoms exhibited before medications were prescribed.

Behavioral or cognitive toxicity—occurs when a medication prevents an adaptive behavior from occurring or impairs cognitive functioning.

Behavioral tolerance—a response that counteracts the behavioral effects of the drug.

Bipolar disorder—a mood disorder characterized by periods of mania (manic episodes) or mild mania (hypomanic episodes) generally alternating with depression. Manic episodes involve at least a weeklong period during which the child has an abnormally elevated or irritable mood.

Bulimia nervosa—an eating disorder characterized by episodes of binge eating that involve eating a very large amount of food in a short period of time (less than 2 hours) and then attempting to prevent weight gain by vomiting, using laxatives, fasting, or exercising excessively.

Central nervous system (CNS)—the brain and spinal cord.

Comorbidity—the co-occurrence of two or more disorders.

Conduct disorder (CD)—a condition characterized by very serious behavior problems that violate the rights of others.

Controlled substances (*see also* Schedule II drugs)—medications with a high potential for abuse and misuse.

Delusions—false beliefs.

Dendrites—branches that extend from the cell body of a neuron and receive information from other neurons.

Depressive disorder—a disorder characterized by a mood episode lasting at least 2 weeks that is marked by symptoms of sadness, irritability, or loss of interest in things the child used to enjoy.

Developmental pediatrician—a pediatrician with expertise in the assessment and clinical management of children with disabilities.

Double-blind studies—experiments where neither the experimenter nor the participants know if the participant is taking an actual medication or a placebo.

Drugs or medications—chemical substances that affect the body. *See* Agents.

Dysthymia—a depressive disorder characterized by a chronically depressed or irritable mood that lasts for more than a year.

Encopresis—an elimination disorder characterized by accidents involving bowel movements that occur at least once per month for 3 months past the age of 4.

Enuresis—an elimination disorder characterized by regular urine accidents after the age of 5. It is typically diagnosed when the child has at least two accidents per week for 3 or more months.

Flat affect—an appearance that shows little emotion.

Generalized anxiety disorder (GAD)—an anxiety disorder characterized by excessive worry about normal, everyday life events.

Half-life—the amount of time it takes for the body to reduce the amount of a drug by about 50%.

Hallucinations—when an individual sees, smells, or hears things that are not there.

Hypomanic episode—similar to a manic episode but lasts for a shorter period and has less severe symptoms.

Interneurons—neurons that send information from one part of the brain to another.

Line graph—a graph with a horizontal line showing time and a vertical line showing amount.

Major depressive episode—*see* Depressive disorder.

Mania—unstable mood characterized by hyperverbal behavior, sleeplessness, pressured speech, elation, and irritability.

Manic episode—mania that lasts at least a week where the child has an abnormally elevated or irritable mood.

Mental retardation—a deficit in intellectual ability and adaptive behaviors that begins before the age of 18 and is characterized by an IQ generally below 70 and deficits in adaptive functioning in two of the following areas: communication, self-care, home living, social or interpersonal skills, use of community resources, self-direction, functional academic skills, work, leisure, health, and safety.

Metabolic tolerance—a physical response that counteracts the effects of medication through metabolic processes.

Motor neurons—neurons that send information to the muscles of the body to make the body move in a desired way.

Multiple drug therapy—multiple medications prescribed to manage polypharmacy or to treat the same disorder.

Neuroleptic malignant syndrome—a rare, extremely serious, potentially fatal reaction from antipsychotic medications. Signs can include confusion, fever, and sweating.

Neuroleptics—*See* Antipsychotic medications.

Neurons—cells in the central nervous system that conduct information between areas of the brain, and between the brain and other parts of the body.

Neurotransmitters—chemicals used to send messages so neurons can "talk" to each other.

Obsessive–compulsive disorder (OCD)—a disruptive behavior disorder classified as an anxiety disorder and characterized by intrusive thoughts or images (obsessions) or impulses (compulsions).

Off-label use—use of a medication for a problem (or in a population) other than that for which it was originally researched and intended.

Oppositional defiant disorder (ODD)—a disruptive behavior disorder characterized by a pattern of defiant behavior that persists over time and across different settings.

Over-the-counter medications—medications available in regular drug stores or grocery stores without a prescription.

Panic disorder—an anxiety disorder characterized by recurrent panic symptoms that are severe enough to warrant the word *attack*, including very intense feelings of fear and symptoms such as sweating, racing heart, shaking, shortness of breath, nausea, dizziness, and chest pain.

Pediatric neurologist—a physician who specializes in diagnosing and treating problems in the brain, spinal cord, muscles, and nervous system in children.

Pediatric or child clinical psychologist—a person who has received intensive training in childhood psychiatric disorders and specializes in the assessment and treatment of developmental, learning, behavioral, and psychiatric problems in children. They have a doctorate degree but cannot prescribe medication.

Pediatric psychiatrist—a medical doctor with expertise in diagnosing and treating psychiatric disorders in children.

Pediatric psychopharmacology—the specific study and application of the effects of medications on the behavior of children.

Pediatrician—a physician who specializes in child health care.

Pervasive developmental disorder not otherwise specified (PDDNOS)—a disorder that has some of the features of Asperger syndrome and autism but does not meet strict diagnostic criteria for those disorders.

Pharmacology—the study of the physical and chemical effects of drugs in the body, the ways in which drugs work, and the effects they have on body chemistry, physiology, and behavior.

Phobia—fear of a specific object or situation, such as heights, small spaces, or spiders.

Placebo—a pill that does not contain any medication but looks like a pill that does.

Placebo effect—the portion of a medication's effectiveness that is due to factors other than the chemical actions of the medication.

Polypharmacy—the concurrent use of multiple medications for multiple problems.

Posttraumatic stress disorder (PTSD)—an anxiety disorder characterized by significant psychological problems following exposure to a life-threatening event such as a car accident, an assault, or a natural disaster.

Psychotic disorder—a disorder characterized by hallucinations or delusions.

Prescription medications—medications prescribed by a physician.

Psychopharmacology—the study of the effects of drugs on psychological processes and behavior.

Psychotropic agents—agents prescribed to alter mood or behavior.

Rebound phenomenon or effect—increased overactivity from baseline levels when a drug wears off.

Reuptake—the process by which a cell takes a released neurotransmitter substance back into itself.

Schedule II drugs (also called controlled substances)—a classification of medications with such a high chance of abuse or addiction that any prescriptions must be handwritten and hand-signed by the physician, and the pharmacist must order the medications on a special blank Drug Enforcement Agency order sheet.

School psychologist—a person with specialized training in psychology and education who provides assessment and intervention for school-age children with developmental, learning, and behavior problems. They may have a master's or doctorate degree but do not prescribe medications.

Selective mutism—a failure to use language in certain situations, usually at school or in public.

Sensory neurons—neurons that conduct information from the outside world (vision, touch, smell) to parts of the brain so that it can be processed.

Separation anxiety disorder—a disorder characterized by severe anxiety about being away from home or being separated from a primary caretaker that persists into early school age.

Soma—the cell body of a neuron.

Substance abuse—a maladaptive pattern of substance use that leads to impairment in life functions, such as failing school, having legal problems, driving while intoxicated, and having interpersonal problems.

Substance dependence—reliance on a drug despite serious, sometimes life-threatening, drug-related problems.

Synapse—the space or cleft between neighboring neurons. Messages are transmitted across these clefts.

Tardive dyskinesia—a serious side effect associated with long-term use of traditional antipsychotics, with symptoms including involuntary movements, particularly involuntary mouth and tongue movements.

Tic—a recurrent movement or vocalization.

Titration—the process of adjusting the dose of a medication until the desired effect is achieved or until adverse effects are observed.

Tolerance—a state that occurs when a dose that previously had an effect on an individual no longer produces the desired effect.

Tourette's disorder (TD)—a disorder characterized by chronic motor and vocal tics.

Withdrawal symptoms—symptoms that occur when a person stops taking a medication.

Appendices

Common Mental Health Medications for Children

Medication			
Generic name	Trade name	Indicated use	Side effects
Antidepressants (atypical)			
Bupropion	Wellbutrin	ADHD	Abdominal pain, agitation, anxiety, constipation, dizziness, dry mouth, excessive sweating, headache, loss of appetite, nausea, palpitations, vomiting, skin rash, sleep disturbances, sore throat, tremor
Mirtazapine	Remeron	Depression	Strange dreams and thoughts, constipation, dizziness, dry mouth, flu-like symptoms, increased appetite, sleepiness, weakness, weight gain
Trazodone	Desyrel	Comorbid ADHD and CD	Dizziness, drowsiness, light-headedness
Venlafaxine	Effexor	Cormorbid ADHD, ODD, and CD	Anxiety, constipation, depression, difficulty breathing, dizziness, dry mouth, itching, loss of appetite, weakness, nausea, nervousness, sedation, skin rash, sleep problems, sweating, tingling hands or feet, tremors, vomiting, strange dreams, weight loss
Antidepressants (serotonin reuptake inhibitors)			
Citalopram	Celessxa	Depression	Abdominal pain, agitation, anxiety, diarrhea, drowsiness, dry mouth, fatigue, indigestion, insomnia, loss of appetite, nausea, sweating, tremor, vomiting
Fluoxetine	Prozac	OCD, panic, separation anxiety, depression	Anxiety, nervousness
Fluvoxamine	Luvox	OCD, panic, separation anxiety, depression	Decreased appetite, constipation, dry mouth, headache, nausea, nervousness, skin rash, sleep problems, sleepiness
Sertraline	Zoloft	OCD, panic, separation anxiety, depression	Diarrhea, dizziness, drowsiness, dry mouth, headache, indigestion, fatigue, insomnia, nausea, nervousness, tingling, or vomiting
Paroxetine	Paxil	OCD, panic, separation anxiety, depression	Constipation or diarrhea, decreased appetite, dizziness, drowsiness, dry mouth, nausea, nervousness, sleeplessness, sweating, tremor, weakness, vertigo

(continued)

Medication			
Generic name	Trade name	Indicated use	Side effects
Antidepressants (tricyclics)			
Amitriptyline	Elavil	Depression	Vision problems, constipation, difficulty urinating, dry mouth, fatigue, sensitivity to sunlight, temperature sensitivity
Clomipramine	Anafranil	OCD, depression	Vision problems, constipation, drowsiness, dry mouth, low blood pressure, nausea, vomiting
Desipramine	Norpramin, Pertofrane	ADHD, depression	Dry mouth, visual disturbance, constipation, dizziness, drowsiness, increased perspiration, mild tremors, insomnia
Imipramine	Tofranil	Depression, enuresis	Dry mouth, constipation, nausea, blurred vision, sedation, stomach upset, nightmares, nervousness, tiredness, convulsions, fainting
Maprotiline	Ludiomil	Depression	Low blood pressure, nervousness, dry mouth, drowsiness
Nortriptyline	Pamelor, Vivactil	Depression	Headache, nausea, sweating, dry mouth, sleepiness or insomnia, diarrhea or constipation, blurry vision, weight gain
Protriptyline	Vivactil	Depression	Headache, nausea, sweating, dry mouth, sleepiness or insomnia, diarrhea or constipation, blurry vision, weight gain
Antihypertensives			
Clonidine	Catapres	PTSD	Sedation, depression, irritability, low blood pressure
Guanfacine	Tenex	Comorbid ADHD and tics	Irritability, tiredness
Nadolol	Corgard	Comorbid ADHD and tics	Sedation, low blood pressure, dry mouth, irritability, depression
Propranolol	Inderal	PTSD, anxiety	Nausea, vomiting, constipation, diarrhea, vivid dreams, depression, dizziness
Antipsychotics (atypical)			
Clozapine	Clozaril	Bipolar symptoms	Drowsiness, dizziness, low blood pressure, increased salivation, racing heartbeat, constipation
Olanzapine	Zyprexa	Reduction of stereotypical and perseverative behaviors	Drowsiness, dry mouth, dizziness, weakness, constipation, upset stomach, increased appetite, mild trembling
Quetiapine	Seroquel	Psychiatric behaviors	Can cause sedation, weight gain, cognitive blunting, decreased seizure threshold; must monitor for movement disorders
Risperidone	Risperdal	Mania	Sleepiness, low blood pressure, dry mouth, blurred vision, constipation, weight gain, difficulty urinating, nasal irritation and stuffiness, stiffness

(continued)

Medication			
Generic name	**Trade name**	**Indicated use**	**Side effects**
Antipsychotics (high potency)			
Haloperidol	Haldol	Psychotic behavior, Tourette's disorder	Akathisia, akinesia, sleepiness, low blood pressure, dry mouth, blurred vision, constipation, weight gain, difficulty urinating, stiffness
Fluphenazine	Prolixin	Psychotic behavior, Tourette's disorder	Akathisia, akinesia, sleepiness, low blood pressure, dry mouth, blurred vision, constipation, weight gain, difficulty urinating, stiffness
Pimozide	Orap	Tourette's disorder	Can cause sedation, weight gain, cognitive blunting, decreased seizure threshold; must monitor for movement disorders
Antipsychotics (low potency)			
Chlorpromazine	Thorazine	Psychotic behavior	Akathisia, akinesia, sleepiness, low blood pressure, dry mouth, blurred vision, constipation, weight gain, difficulty urinating, stiffness
Mesoridazine	Serentil	Psychotic behavior	Akathisia, akinesia, sleepiness, low blood pressure, dry mouth, blurred vision, constipation, weight gain, difficulty urinating, stiffness
Molindone	Moban	Psychotic behavior	Weight gain
Thioridazine	Mellaril	Schizophrenia	Sleepiness, low blood pressure, dry mouth, blurred vision, constipation, weight gain, difficulty urinating, stiffness
Antipsychotics (medium potency)			
Loxapine	Loxitane	Schizophrenia	Can cause sedation, weight gain, cognitive blunting, decreased seizure threshold; must monitor for movement disorders
Perphenazine	Trilafon	Psychotic disorders	Motor movements
Thiothixene	Navane	Schizophrenia	Sleepiness, low blood pressure, dry mouth, blurred vision, constipation, weight gain, difficulty urinating, stiffness, cognitive blunting, decreased seizure threshold
Trifluoperazine	Stelazine	Psychotic behavior	Drowsiness, motor restlessness, muscle spasms, movement disorders

(continued)

Common Mental Health Medications for Children

Medication			
Generic name	**Trade name**	**Indicated use**	**Side effects**
Anxiety-breaking agents (anxiolytics)			
Antihistamines			
Chlorpheniramine	Chlor-Trimeton	Anxiety, sleep disorder	Sedation, cognitive impairment, anticholinergic (dry mouth), constipation, blurred vision
Diphenhydramine	Benadryl	Anxiety, sleep disorder	Sedation, cognitive impairment, anticholinergic (dry mouth), constipation, blurred vision
Hydroxyzine	Vistaril, Atarax	Anziety, sleep disorder	Sedation, cognitive impairment, anticholinergic (dry mouth), constipation, blurred vision
Atypical			
Buspirone	Buspar	GAD, social phobia, panic disorder, separation anxiety disorder	Can cause dizziness, confusion, disinhibition and drowsiness
Benzodiazepines (partial list)			
Alprazolam	Xanax	Anxiety	Clumsiness, sleepiness
Chlordiazepoxide	Librium	Anxiety	Clumsiness, sleepiness
Clonazepam	Klonopin	GAD, panic disorder, separation anxiety	Anxiety, behavior problems, insomnia, irritability, drowsiness, problems with coordination
Clorazepate	Tranxene	Anxiety	Clumsiness, sleepiness
Diazepam	Valium	Anxiety, agitation	Clumsiness, sleepiness
Lorazepam	Ativan	Anxiety, agitation	Clumsiness, dizziness, sleepiness, unsteadiness, weakness
Oxazepam	Serax	Anxiety	Mild drowsiness, skin rashes
Triazolam	Halcion	Insomnia	Clumsiness, sleepiness
Monamine oxidase inhibitors			
Phenelzine	Nardil	Atypical depression	Dizziness, headaches, sleep problems
Tranylcypromine	Parnate	Atypical depression	Hypertensive crisis

(continued)

Common Mental Health Medications for Children (*page 5 of 5*)

Medication			
Generic name	**Trade name**	**Indicated use**	**Side effects**
Mood stabilizers			
Carbamazepine	Tegretol	Mania	Dizziness, drowsiness, nausea, blurred vision
Gabapentin	Neurontin		Fatigue, dizziness
Lamotrigine	Lamictal		Fatigue, rashes, dizziness, blurred or double vision
Lithium salts	Lithobid, Lithonate, Lithotabs, Eskalith, Cibalith	Mania	Diarrhea, frequent urination, nausea, skin rashes, tremor, weight gain
Tiagabine	Gabitril		Fatigue, dizziness, unstable walking, associated with risk of seizures in patients without epilepsy treated off label
Topiramate	Topamax	Bipolar disorder, seizure disorder	Fatigue, dizziness, nervousness, tingling in extremities
Valproic acid	Valproate, Depakote, Depakene sprinkles	Mania	Cramps, stomach upset, diarrhea, indigestion, drowsiness, dizziness, lethargy (watch for liver problems)
Stimulants			
Amphetamine	Biphetamine	ADHD	Can cause appetite suppression, insomnia, dizziness, gastrointestinal problems and irritability, emotional ups and downs
Amphetamine compounds	Adderall	ADHD	
Dextroamphetamine	Dexedrine	ADHD	Restlessness, constipation or diarrhea, dizziness, dry mouth, headache, heart palpitations, high blood pressure, decreased appetite, sleeplessness, stomach and intestinal disturbances, tremors, unpleasant taste in the mouth, weight loss
Magnesium pemoline	Cylert	ADHD	Insomnia, depression, dizziness, drowsiness, headache, irritability, tics, decreased appetite, mild depression, nausea, liver problems (rarely)
Methamphetamine	Desoxyn	ADHD	Sleep problems, nervousness, decreased appetite, abdominal pain, weight loss, sleep problems, fast heartbeat
Methylphenidate	Ritalin	ADHD	Sleep problems, nervousness, decreased appetite, abdominal pain, weight loss, sleep problems, fast heartbeat

Event Observation Log

Child's name: _____   Teacher's name: _____

Week of: _____

Date	Time	Event

Appendix 3

Letter to Physician

As _____'s teacher, I have been asked to provide the following information about school-related issues and progress.

Child's name: _____ Child's grade: _____

Form completed by: _____ Position: _____

Type of classroom: _____ School: _____

Telephone: _____ Best times to call: _____

This child's academic difficulties include:

This child's academic strengths include:

This child's behavioral difficulties include:

This child's behavioral strengths include:

Does this child have friends? Describe any social difficulties or problems.

(continued)

Describe any unusual behaviors.

Is this child absent often? YES NO If yes, for what reason(s)?

Questions and concerns about this child:

Attach work sample, report card, and behavior observations to this form.

Ranking Problem Behaviors

Child's name: _____   Date of report: _____

WHICH OF THIS CHILD'S BEHAVIORS CONCERN YOU MOST?

Please rank the problem behaviors that are of most concern to you. Place a 1 next to the behavior that is of most concern, a 2 next to the behavior that is your next concern, and so on. For example, if you are most concerned about tics but also concerned about hyperactivity, you would mark a 1 next to tics and a 2 next to hyperactivity. If a behavior is not a problem for this child, leave it blank.

_____ Aggression (hitting, kicking, biting)

_____ Compulsions (certain things the child feels he or she must do)

_____ Delusions (bizarre beliefs that are inappropriate for the child's developmental stage)

_____ Emotional outbursts

_____ Emotional ups and downs and mood swings

_____ Hair pulling

_____ Hallucinations (seeing or hearing things that are not there)

_____ Hyperactivity

_____ Impulsivity (doing things without thinking)

_____ Inattention or lack of focus

_____ Lack of emotional expression (also known as a flat affect)

_____ Nervousness, anxiety, worrying

_____ Obsessions (can't stop thinking about certain things, disturbing ideas)

_____ Repetitive motor behaviors (flapping, rocking)

_____ Self-injurious behaviors (head banging, face slapping)

_____ Tearfulness, sadness

_____ Tics

_____ Withdrawn behaviors (not talking to others, being alone)

Appendix 5

Proper Handling Procedures for Medications for Children

- Keep medications in a secure place in clearly labeled bottles.

- Keep medication in its original child-proof bottle, labeled with the child's name.

- Dispense medication as written on the bottle or elsewhere by the child's physicians. Require a note from the physician if the dosage or times are changed.

- Keep a log of medication administrations so that each pill in a bottle can be accounted for. The physician may provide this log or you can use the one found in Appendix 8.

- Some children may be sensitive about taking medication at school. Talk to them and their parents about how they would like you to handle the subject with the other children in the class.

- Make a plan that details what to do if a child misses a dose of medication.

- Have phone numbers of the child's parents (home, work, and cell phones) and a specific person or persons accessible in case of emergency.

- Drugs and alcohol can change the way some medications affect the child. Alert parents immediately if you suspect a child is using drugs or alcohol. Your school likely has a policy about this.

- Refrigerate liquids as required because most liquids lose strength if stored at room temperature.

- Measure medication using a marked medication cup, dropper, or spoon. An ordinary teaspoon is not accurate.

Medication Initiation Form

Child's name: _____   Date of report: _____

Medication: _____   Dosage: _____

Time of administration: _____

1. If the medication is to be given at school, what time does it need to be given?

2. How close to the assigned time must the medication be given? For example, if we are taking a timed test, can your child take her medication later in the day?

3. What should we do if a dose is missed?

4. Might your child resist taking medication? What should we do if your child refuses to take the medication? Might your child pretend to take it but spit it out later?

5. What are signs of overdose of this medication?

(continued)

6. What are some common side effects that we might need to look out for? Which side effects are potentially dangerous?

7. Does the child need to take the medication with food?

8. Did your physician ask us to complete any forms about your child's learning and behavior?

Appendix 7

Authorization to Administer Medication

I authorize designated agents of (school name) _____
to administer the following medication to my child, _____.

My child's health care provider is _____. Telephone _____.

My child's condition is

_____.

The purpose of this medication is

_____.

Name of medication: _____

Method of administration: _____. Times of administration: _____.

Possible side effects: _____

_____

In case of emergency, contact _____ Telephone _____

or _____ Telephone _____

I agree to indemnify and hold harmless this school, their agents, and servants against all claims as a result of any and all acts performed under this authority.

Parent/guardian signature: _____ Date: _____

Parent/guardian name (please print): _____

Parent/guardian telephone: _____

Witness signature: _____

Appendix 8

Monthly Medication Log

Important: Use a new log for each bottle of medication. If the child takes two or more medications, use separate logs.

Child's name: _____ Month: _____

Medication: _____ Amount provided: _____

Date medication received: _____

Time to give first dose: _____ Dose amount: _____

Time to give second dose: _____ Dose amount: _____

Day	Date	Time administered	Staff initials	Time administered	Staff initials
Monday					
Tuesday					
Wednesday					
Thursday					
Friday					
Monday					
Tuesday					
Wednesday					
Thursday					
Friday					
Monday					
Tuesday					
Wednesday					
Thursday					
Friday					
Monday					
Tuesday					
Wednesday					
Thursday					
Friday					

Appendix 9

Medication Contract

I, _____, agree to take my medication every day
at _____ A.M./P.M.

I will earn 1 point each time I take my medication.

When I earn _____ points, I will receive

_____.

Child's signature: _____

Parent's signature: _____
School personnel signature: _____

FDA Black Box Warnings for Antidepressants

Suicidality in Children and Adolescents

Antidepressants increase the risk of suicidal thinking and behavior (suicidality) in children and adolescents with major depressive disorder (MDD) and other psychiatric disorders. Anyone considering the use of [Drug Name] or any other antidepressant in a child or adolescent must balance this risk with the clinical need. Patients who are started on therapy should be observed closely for clinical worsening, suicidality, or unusual changes in behavior. Families and caregivers should be advised of the need for close observation and communication with the prescriber. [Drug Name] is not approved for use in pediatric patients except for patients with [Any approved pediatric claims here]. (See Warnings and Precautions: Pediatric Use)

Pooled analyses of short-term (4 to 16 weeks) placebo-controlled trials of nine antidepressant drugs (SSRIs and others) in children and adolescents with MDD, obsessive compulsive disorder (OCD), or other psychiatric disorders (a total of 24 trials involving over 4400 patients) have revealed a greater risk of adverse events representing suicidal thinking or behavior (suicidality) during the first few months of treatment in those receiving antidepressants. The average risk of such events on drug was 4%, twice the placebo risk of 2%. No suicides occurred in these trials.

These antidepressants currently on the market (as of February 3, 2005) carry the warning labels:

- Anafranil (clomipramine HCl)
- Asendin (amoxapine)
- Aventyl (nortriptyline HCl)
- Celexa (citalopram HBr)
- Cymbalta (duloxetine HCl)
- Desyrel (trazodone HCl)
- Effexor (venlafaxine HCl)
- Elavil (amitriptyline HCl)
- Etrafon (perphenazine/amitriptyline)
- Lexapro (escitalopram oxalate)
- Limbitrol (chlordiazepoxide/amitriptyline)
- Ludiomil (maprotiline HCl)
- Luvox (fluvoxamine maleate)
- Marplan (isocarboxazid)
- Nardil (phenelzine sulfate)
- Norpramin (desipramine HCl)
- Pamelor (nortriptyline HCl)
- Parnate (tranylcypromine sulfate)
- Paxil (paroxetine HCl)
- Pexeva (paroxetine mesylate)
- Prozac (fluoxetine HCl)
- Remeron (mirtazapine)
- Sarafem (fluoxetine HCl)
- Serzone (nefazodone HCl)
- Sinequan (doxepin HCl)
- Surmontil (trimipramine)
- Symbyax (olanzapine/fluoxetine)
- Tofranil (imipramine HCl)
- Tofranil-PM (imipramine pamoate)
- Triavil (perphenazine/amitriptyline)
- Vivactil (protriptyline HCl)
- Wellbutrin (bupropion HCl)
- Zoloft (sertraline HCl)
- Zyban (bupropion HCl)

Behavior Observation Form 1: Event Recording

1. Use this form to record how often behaviors occur during a specific time period.
2. The length of the observation should be about the same each day. For behaviors that happen often (out of seat, talking without raising hand), a short observation period (5 minutes) may be enough. For behaviors that don't happen often (hitting, biting), a longer period of an hour or more may work better.
3. You can chose to track one behavior or two behaviors. Make sure behaviors are specific.

Behavior 1: _____

Behavior 2: _____

Date	Observation start time	Observation end time	Behavior 1	Behavior 2

Behavior Observation Form 2: Duration Recording

Use this form to record how long a behavior lasts. Track only one behavior with this form. Use a second form to track a different behavior.

Behavior: _____

Date	Time behavior started	Time behavior ended	Duration (minutes)

Behavior Observation Form 3: Total Duration Recording

Use this form to record how much time a child spends engaged in a certain behavior. Track one behavior with this form. Use a second form to track a different behavior.

Behavior: _____

Date	Total time of observation	Total time engaged in target behavior (minutes)

Appendix 14

Line Graph 1: Less Frequent Behaviors

1. Use this graph to keep track of behaviors that happen less often (from zero to 20 times in an observation period).
2. Write a title for the graph (e.g., Number of Times Claire Hit Her Hand on Her Desk during Speech Class).
3. Make a dot for each day or session for which you have data. For example, if the child completed six math problems during the first session, place a dot on the line above 1 and next to 6.
4. Connect the dots.

Title: _____

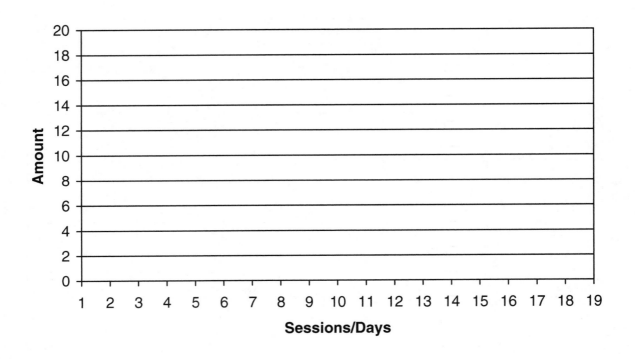

Line Graph 2: More Frequent Behaviors and Percentages

1. Use this graph to keep track of behaviors that happen more often (from 20 to 100 times in an observation period) or to keep track of percentages
2. Write a title for the graph (e.g., Number of Times Claire Hit Her Hand on Her Desk during Speech Class).
3. Make a dot for each day or session for which you have data. For example, if the child completed five math problems during the first session, place a dot on the line halfway between 0 and 10.
4. Connect the dots.

Title: _____

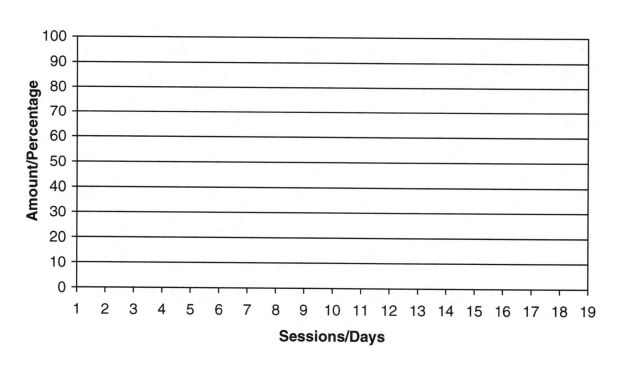

Appendix 16

Side Effects

Have you noticed any of the following behaviors in the past week? Check each one noticed.

☐ Sleepy/sedated

☐ Hyperactive

☐ Very thirsty

☐ Going to the bathroom a lot

☐ "Out of it" or "like a zombie"

☐ Headaches

☐ Concentration problems

☐ Memory problems

☐ Sadness

☐ Crying a lot

☐ Sleeping at school

☐ Flat: no emotions

☐ Tremor

☐ Tics

☐ Toileting accidents

☐ Nausea, vomiting, stomach problems

☐ Sweating excessively

☐ Turning very red

☐ Complaining of dizziness

☐ Sensitivity to light

☐ Staring blankly

☐ Not eating

☐ Irritability

☐ Nervousness

☐ Restlessness

☐ Tongue/mouth movements

☐ Excessive talking

☐ Unmotivated

☐ Blurry vision

☐ Drooling

Index